HARDCORE Pharmacology

Rodrigo E. Saenz, MD
Internal Medicine Resident
Louisiana State University Medical Center
New Orleans, Louisiana

Benjamin W. Sears, MD
Orthopaedic Surgery Resident
Loyola University Medical Center
Chicago, Illinois

Paul Adam Dabisch, PhD
Operational Toxicology Team
United States Army Edgewood Chemical Biological Center
Aberdeen Proving Ground, Maryland

 Lippincott Williams & Wilkins
a Wolters Kluwer business

Philadelphia · Baltimore · New York · London
Buenos Aires · Hong Kong · Sydney · Tokyo

Acquisitions Editor: Beverly Copland
Development Editor: Kate Heinle
Production Editor: Jennifer Kowalewski
Interior Designer: Janice Bielawa
Cover Designer: Shawn Girsberger
Compositor: Graphicraft Ltd in Hong Kong
Printer: Walsworth

351 West Camden Street
Baltimore, MD 21201

530 Walnut Street
Philadelphia, PA 19106

The publisher is not responsible (as a matter of product liability, negligence, or
otherwise) for any injury resulting from any material contained herein. This publication
contains information relating to general principles of medical care that should not be
construed as specific instructions for individual patients. Manufacturers' product information
and package inserts should be reviewed for current information, including contraindications,
dosages, and precautions.

Printed in the United States of America

Library of Congress Cataloging-in-Publication Data

Saenz, Rodrigo E.
   Hardcore pharmacology / Rodrigo E. Saenz, Benjamin W. Sears,
Paul Adam Dabisch.
    p. ; cm.
  ISBN-13: 978-1-4051-0454-8 (pbk. : alk. paper)
  ISBN-10: 1-4051-0454-6 (pbk. : alk. paper)
    1. Pharmacology—Outlines, syllabi, etc. 2. Pharmacology—Examinations, questions, etc.
I. Sears, Benjamin W. II. Dabisch, Paul Adam. III. Title.
  [DNLM: 1. Pharmacology—Examination Questions. 2. Pharmacology—
Outlines. QV 18.2 S127h 2006]
  RM301.14.S24 2006
  615'.1'076—dc22

2005010315

*The publishers have made every effort to trace the copyright holders for borrowed material. If they
have inadvertently overlooked any, they will be pleased to make the necessary arrangements at the
first opportunity.*

To purchase additional copies of this book, call our customer service department at
(800) 638-3030 or fax orders to **(301) 223-2320**. International customers should call
(301) 223-2300.

Visit Lippincott Williams & Wilkins on the Internet: http://www.LWW.com. Lippincott
Williams & Wilkins customer service representatives are available from 8:30 am to
6:00 pm, EST.

05 06 07 08 09
1 2 3 4 5 6 7 8 9 10

To our families, friends and loved ones who have supported us selflessly
and unquestionably throughout the pursuit of our dreams
&
To all MS IIs, there is a light at the end of the tunnel.

About the Authors

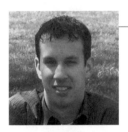

Paul Adam Dabisch

Paul Dabisch is a research biologist at the US Army's Edgewood Chemical Biological Center. He has a Ph.D. in pharmacology from Tulane University in New Orleans, and B.S. in crop sciences from the University of Illinois at Urbana-Champaign. He also holds the rank of First Lieutenant in the US Army Reserve, and is currently assigned to the 2290th US Army Hospital at Walter Reed Army Medical Center.

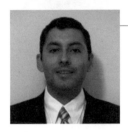

Rodrigo E. Saenz

Rodrigo Saenz was born in Panama City, Panama in 1977. He completed college with a Bachelor of Science degree in Biology from the University of Louisiana at Lafayette in 1998 and a Master of Science in Pharmacology from Tulane University in 2001. Rodrigo will graduate from Louisiana State University Health Sciences Center School of Medicine in New Orleans with a Medical Doctorate degree in May 2005 and will go on to start an Internal Medicine Residency at the LSU Medical Center of Louisiana in New Orleans in July 2005.

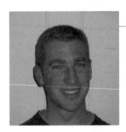

Benjamin W. Sears

Ben Sears was born in Fort Collins, Colorado in 1977, growing up in Aurora, Colorado before attending Colorado State University in Fort Collins. In 2000, he graduated from CSU with a Bachelor of Science in Zoology and a Minor in Nutrition. In 2001, he earned a Master of Science in Pharmacology from Tulane University in New Orleans, Louisiana. Ben will graduate from Loyola University Chicago, Stritch School of Medicine with a Medical Doctorate degree in June, 2005 and will start an Orthopaedic Surgery residency at Loyola University Medical Center, Chicago in July 2005.

A Note to the Reader

The concept of **HARDCORE** *Pharmacology* was born on a dark, rainy day in a small coffee shop in the city of New Orleans. As second-year medical students struggling to sort through the ridiculous amount of medical information tested by Step 1 of the USMLE, we were struck by the lack of easily readable and high-yield pharmacology texts available to students. We were unable to find one good source that provided us with a comprehensive, easy-to-understand review of pharmacology, and it took considerable effort on our part to sift through the copious amount of pharmacology information available in order to identify and master the information that would be tested on Step 1. Even the books which were supposed to be high-yield had too much information—**we needed something which that was pared down to just the most heavily-tested, "hardcore" facts.**

GETTING HARDCORE

As we scoured countless "high-yield" books and completed thousands of review questions, we began to recognize a distinct and consistent pattern in the type of information tested on the pharmacology section of the board exam. Immediately after completing Step 1, we knew that our intuition was right and that, **by focusing primarily on three "hardcore" concepts: drug indications, mechanism of action, and side effects, we were able to correctly answer the vast majority of the pharmacology questions on USMLE Step 1.** We also discovered a lack of student resources that covered the less traditional, but still key, concepts tested by the board exam, including toxicology, drug allergies, teratogenic drugs (drugs that can be safely used during pregnancy and when breast-feeding), and cytochrome P-450 drug inducers and inhibitors. In addition, the board exam includes questions involving figures and graphs, often complex in appearance, that can be intimidating to students who have had limited practice with such questions.

Our pharmacology backgrounds and recent Step 1 experience came together to develop this ultra high-yield pharmacology review **book that brings you the information that is actually tested on the board exam.** And that's how the idea for **HARDCORE** *Pharmacology* was started. The enthusiastic feedback we've gotten from student reviewers encouraged us to expand the **HARDCORE** series: **HARDCORE** *Neuroscience*, **HARDCORE** *Pathology*, and **HARDCORE** *Microbiology and Immunology* are already in the works, with more to come.

FORMATTING AND SPECIAL FEATURES

On top of being concise and high-yield, we wanted to make this book fun and easy to use. Throughout the text we have broken out commonly tested pharmacological principles and critical concepts into hardcore boxes for rapid review—if you don't remember anything else, remember those!

To help make the page easier to skim quickly, the major drugs in each class are indicated by this icon 🔫 and in Chapter 10, the Hardcore bug targets are signified with this icon ⊕. Buzzwords, key terms, mnemonics and formulas are bolded in the text for additional emphasis.

The book has been organized by systems to closely represent the content of Step 1, with special chapters devoted to covering chemotherapeutics, antimicrobials, antifungals, antimycobaterials, antivirals, and antiparasitic drugs, and well as toxicology. Hardcore Reviews at the end of most chapters provide comprehensive high-yield tables for a quick summary. Finally, to allow for even more Step 1 practice, a chapter containing 25 board-format Q&As has been added based on the helpful feedback from our reviewers.

We also included 2 chapters specifically covering the highly-tested, less-traditional concepts (Hardcore Board Concepts) that are not included in most review texts, as well as a chapter composed of board-style figures and graphs with review questions and answers (Hardcore Figures and Graphs). We believe that by mastering these concepts you can significantly enhance your Step 1 score.

The **HARDCORE** series is for students taking Step 1, written by students who have recently taken Step 1, and **HARDCORE** *Pharmacology* is designed for students with limited time to review the concepts of medical pharmacology tested on USMLE Step 1. We believe this is one of the most hardcore, high-yield, yet comprehensive pharmacology review books available, and we hope that you find this text as useful as we believe it would have been to us while preparing to take Step 1.

Rodrigo E. Saenz
Benjamin W. Sears
Paul A. Dabisch

Contributors

Timothy T. Belski
Graduate Student
Johns Hopkins University
Baltimore, Maryland

David V. Daniels, MD
Internal Medicine Resident
Stanford University Hospitals
Palo Alto, California

Lisa M. Spear, MD
Emergency Medicine Resident
University of Illinois at Chicago
Chicago, Illinois

Reviewers

Luther Adair, II
Class of 2006
Meharry Medical College
Nashville, Tennessee

Ruben Cohen
Class of 2007
Louisiana State University Health Sciences Center
New Orleans, Louisiana

Landon Colling
Class of 2006
Southern Illinois University School of Medicine
Springfield, Illinois

Jessica Flynn
Class of 2006
Johns Hopkins University School of Medicine
Baltimore, Maryland

Jae Lim
Class of 2007
Brown Medical School
Providence, Rhode Island

Frederick Shieh
Class of 2006
Boston University School of Medicine
Boston, Massachusetts

Jeremy B. Wingard
Class of 2006
Duke University School of Medicine
Durham, North Carolina

Jennifer Zile
Class of 2006
Medical College of South Carolina
Charleston, South Carolina

Acknowledgments

This book would have never been made possible without the contributions and criticism of several very important people. We would like to thank Lisa Spear from Loyola Medical School Chicago, Stritch School of Medicine, Class of 2005 for her eagle-eyed editing skills and creative mnemonics that acted as a catalyst for us to even consider writing this book proposal. We would also like to thank David Daniels and Jim Prahl, both from Loyola Chicago class of 2005, for their suggestions and insight into key components of this text.

Thanks Dr. Rolando Saenz, Professor of Medicine, School of Medicine University Medical Center, Lafayette, LA for his critique and review of the Antimicrobial and Antifungal, Mycobacterium, Viruses, and Parasites chapters.

Thanks to Tim Birch of San Diego, John Liles and Tracy Taylor, both from New Orleans, for in-depth research that contributed to this book.

Thanks to our original publisher, Blackwell Publishing, especially Beverly Copland, and our current publisher Lippincott Williams & Wilkins, for taking a chance on three unknown students with an idea, and guiding us through the production of both this book and the entire Hardcore Series. Both publishing companies and staff have been extremely enthusiastic, positive and dedicated to this series and has made this process easy and enjoyable to complete. Also, we would like to thank Kate Heinle for assisting us with the technical and procedural aspects of bringing a manuscript into print.

Rodrigo E. Saenz
Benjamin W. Sears
Paul A. Dabisch

Table of Contents

CHAPTER 1

Principles of Pharmacology

PHARMACOKINETICS

Pharmacokinetics refers to the study of the processes of absorption, distribution, biotransformation, and excretion of drugs within the body.

Factors affecting the concentration of drug at its site of action:

- Amount of drug administered (dose)
- Rate of absorption, which is affected by:
  - Physicochemical properties of the drug (i.e., solubility, degree of ionization, molecular weight)
  - Concentration of the drug at the site of absorption
  - Amount of blood flow to the site of absorption
  - Surface area for absorption

Bioavailability

The amount of drug reaching the systemic circulation unchanged following administration. The bioavailability of a drug can be quantified from the graph of plasma concentration versus time (Figure 1-1).

Tracing A (solid line) shows the plasma concentration versus time for a drug given intravenously (IV). Tracing B (dashed line) shows the plasma concentration versus time for the same drug given by another route of administration, "X." The bioavailability of a dose of drug administered by route X can be quantified using the following formula:

$$\text{Bioavailability} = AUC_{\text{Route X}} / AUC_{IV}$$

AUC = Area under the concentration-versus-time curve for a particular route of administration

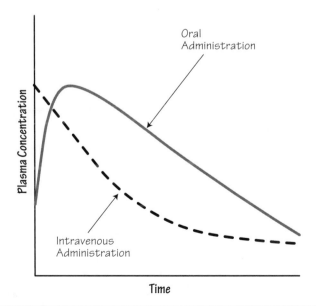

Figure 1-1 Plasma concentration versus time tracings for a drug administered by two different routes. Notice that the peak plasma concentration following oral administration occurs later than for intravenous administration due to absorption from the gastrointestinal tract and distribution. Notice that intravenous administration does not have a distribution phase and, thus, the peak plasma concentration occurs at time 0.

Notice that the bioavailability of a drug given IV is 1, meaning that all of the administered drug reaches the systemic circulation and is available to the target tissue. Drugs administered enterally generally have a bioavailability less than 1 due to:

- Incomplete absorption from the gastrointestinal tract
- First-pass effect in the liver
- Drug distribution to and binding in tissue
- Biotransformation and excretion of the drug

Routes of Administration

There are two routes of administration:

1) Enteral Administration

The administration of a drug by a route involving the alimentary canal, including oral, rectal, and sublingual administration.

- *Advantages*:   – Easy administration
                   – Convenient
- *Disadvantages*:   – Variable rate of absorption between drugs
                      – First-pass effect (see below)

FIRST-PASS EFFECT

Drugs absorbed from the digestive tract enter the portal circulation and pass through the liver before entering the systemic circulation. Therefore, the bioavailability of drugs metabolized by the liver can be reduced when administered orally. This is commonly referred to as the ***first-pass effect*** or ***first-pass metabolism***.

2) Parenteral Administration

The administration of a drug by a route not involving the digestive tract, including:

- Intravenous (IV)
- Subcutaneous (SC)
- Intramuscular (IM)
- Intra-arterial (IA)
- Intrathecal (IT)
- Intraperitoneal (IP)
- Inhaled (IH)

Biotransformation and Metabolism

Types of Biotransformation Reactions

The two major types of biotransformation reactions are defined as follows:

1) Phase I Reactions—Expose or introduce functional groups (commonly –OH, –NH$_2$, or –SH$_2$ groups) on a drug in an attempt to make the compound more water soluble.

- These reactions result in a small increase in the water solubility of a drug, which can enhance excretion.
- Phase I reactions make a drug more susceptible to phase II reactions.
- The majority of phase I reactions are catalyzed by hepatic cytochrome P450 enzymes.
- These reactions can result in the loss of the pharmacologic activity of a drug.

2) Phase II Reactions—Conjugation reactions involving the formation of a covalent bond between the drug molecule and highly polar molecules such as acetate, sulfate, and glucuronic acid. This polar conjugate is highly water soluble and is readily excreted from the body in the urine. These reactions may or may not be preceded by a phase I reaction and, like phase I reactions, often result in the loss of the pharmacologic activity of the drug.

Rate of Biotransformation

Can be affected by:

- **Induction** of the biotransformation pathway, resulting in enhanced metabolism of the drug
- **Inhibition** of the biotransformation pathway, prolonging the duration of effect of the drug
- **Genetic differences** among individuals. This is often referred to as ***pharmacogenomics***.

Routes of Excretion

- **Urine**—Drugs filtered or secreted into the kidney are excreted in the urine. This is the major route of elimination for most drugs.

HARDCORE

A significant first-pass effect may also occur in the lungs and the skin for drugs administered via inhalation and transdermally, respectively.

HARDCORE

Most biotransformation reactions are enzymatic and occur in the liver, although all tissues possess some metabolic capacity.

HARDCORE

A genetic polymorphism is a hereditary variant that occurs in more than 1% of the population being studied.

- **Feces**—Many hepatic metabolites of drugs are secreted via the bile into the intestinal tract. The metabolites are then excreted in the feces. However, some of the metabolites may be reabsorbed into the bloodstream, referred to as *enterohepatic recirculation*, and ultimately be eliminated by the kidneys.
- **Expired air**—Expired air from the lungs may be a route of excretion for compounds that are in a gaseous state at room temperature.
- **Breast milk**—Lipophilic and basic compounds can be excreted in breast milk and, thus, have the potential to be passed on to offspring.
- **Sweat and saliva**—This is a minor route of excretion. Drugs excreted in the sweat can cause dermatitis. Drugs excreted in the saliva can be swallowed and reabsorbed in the gastrointestinal tract.

Pharmacokinetic Parameters

Apparent Volume of Distribution

The **apparent volume of distribution** is used to describe the distribution of the chemical throughout the body based on the dose of a drug given and the measured plasma concentration of the drug.

Factors that can affect the volume of distribution include:

- Degree of plasma protein binding of the drug
- Physicochemical properties of the drug (e.g., lipophilicity, pK_a, etc.)
- Age and body composition of the patient
- Gender of the patient
- Any diseases present in the patient

The phrase "apparent volume of distribution" is used instead of just "volume of distribution" because the calculated volume is not always physiologically reasonable (see below). The apparent volume of distribution (V_D) can be calculated using the following formula:

$$V_D = \text{Loading dose} / C_o$$

Loading dose = The first dose of a drug administered. Its purpose is to rapidly achieve a therapeutic concentration of drug in the plasma.

C_o = The **initial concentration** of drug measured in a reference body fluid, usually plasma, following distribution

TWO EXAMPLES OF VOLUME OF DISTRIBUTION

Example 1: Ibuprofen has a V_D of 0.15 liters per kilogram of body weight
For a 70-kg man, $V_D = 10.5$ L

Example 2: Fluoxetine has a V_D of 35 liters per kilogram of body weight
For a 70-kg man, $V_D = 2450$ L

For some drugs, such as ibuprofen, the calculated apparent volume of distribution is reasonable. For other drugs, such as fluoxetine, the result of the calculation may seem ridiculous. Recall that the total body water of a 70-kg man is only around 42 L; so how is it possible that the fluoxetine has apparently distributed to 2450 L? The answer: it hasn't. (This is the reason for the word "apparent.") So what does it mean when the calculated apparent volume of distribution is greater than the total body water? Remember that we are measuring the concentration of the drug only in a reference body fluid (usually the plasma compartment), not the whole body. If the calculated apparent volume of distribution is much larger than the total body water, it means that the drug is rapidly distributing to compartments and tissues other than the plasma compartment, reducing the amount of drug initially measured in the plasma (i.e., C_o).

Elimination Clearance

The volume of plasma cleared of drug per unit time; thus, its units describe flow rate (i.e., mL/min). Elimination clearance can occur in several organs, including the kidneys, liver, and lungs.

TOTAL CLEARANCE

This is the total sum of all involved organ clearances for a particular drug.

CLEARANCE (CL)

Clearance of a drug can be calculated from the following formula:

$$CL = \text{Rate of elimination} / C_{rf}$$

C_{rf} = The concentration of the drug in a reference fluid, such as plasma

MAINTENANCE DOSING RATE

This is the amount of a drug that must be given per unit time to maintain a desired concentration

HARDCORE

The loading dose is usually given intravenously, since this is the route of administration with the most rapid distribution phase.

HARDCORE

The elimination clearance in a particular organ cannot be greater than the blood flow to that organ.

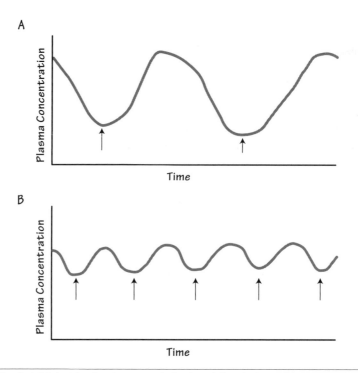

Figure 1-2 The effect of dosing interval on plasma concentration. Arrows indicate the time at which a dose was given. **(A)** Plasma concentrations for a drug given at a longer dose interval. **(B)** Plasma concentrations for a drug given at a shorter dose interval. Notice that a shorter dosing interval results in less variation in the plasma concentration even though the mean plasma concentration may be the same in each case.

in a reference body fluid. Ideally, the rate of administration should equal the rate of elimination, resulting in a steady concentration of drug in the blood. In reality, it is not possible to match the rate of administration and the rate of elimination continuously, because metabolism is a continuous process, while drug administration is usually intermittent (except for IV infusion). This results in fluctuation in the plasma concentration of the drug (Figure 1-2).

STEADY STATE CONCENTRATION (C_{ss})

The C_{ss} is the concentration at which the amount of drug eliminated for a dosing interval equals the dose given for that interval. It is a function of both the maintenance dosing rate and the clearance (CL). The steady state concentration of a drug can be estimated using the following formula:

$$C_{ss} = \text{Maintenance dosing rate / CL}$$

FIRST-ORDER ELIMINATION KINETICS

For a drug eliminated according to first-order kinetics, the elimination is proportional to the plasma concentration. Therefore, a **constant _fraction_** of the drug is eliminated per unit of time (Figure 1-3A).

ZERO-ORDER ELIMINATION KINETICS

For a drug eliminated according to zero-order kinetics, a **constant _amount_** of the drug is eliminated per unit of time (Figure 1-3B). Zero-order kinetics occur when the elimination mechanism for a drug becomes saturated.

HARDCORE

Drugs cleared by zero-order kinetics include *aspirin*, *phenytoin*, and *ethanol*.

HARDCORE

Drugs eliminated according to zero-order kinetics will eventually follow first-order elimination kinetics when enough of the drug is eliminated and the elimination mechanism is no longer saturated.

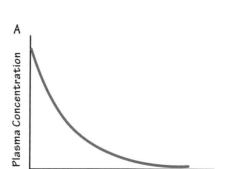
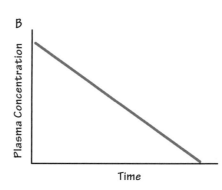

Figure 1-3 **(A)** Plasma concentration versus time for a drug eliminated via first-order kinetics. **(B)** Plasma concentration versus time for a drug eliminated via zero-order kinetics.

ELIMINATION HALF-LIFE

The **elimination half-life** is the amount of time required to eliminate 50% of the body's content of a drug. Factors affecting the half-life of a drug include:

- The rate of elimination clearance
- The degree of plasma protein binding
- The age and body composition of the patient

The following formula can be used to estimate the elimination half-life of a drug:

$$T_{1/2} = 0.69 \, V_D \, / \, CL$$

HARDCORE

Drugs infused at a constant rate will reach steady state after approximately *four to five half-lives*.

PHARMACODYNAMICS

Pharmacodynamics is the study of the physiological and biochemical effects of drugs on the body, including their mechanisms of action and the relationship between drug concentration and the observed effect.

Receptor-Ligand Interactions

Receptors

A receptor is a macromolecular structure, usually located within a cell or on the surface of a cell, characterized by selective binding of a specific substance and a specific physiologic effect that accompanies the binding. Receptors are most commonly proteins, although other cellular components, such as nucleic acids, can also act as receptors.

Be aware that some texts, including this one, define a receptor to be a macromolecule. Given this limitation, there are drugs that act by nonreceptor-mediated mechanisms. For example, an *antacid* would neutralize stomach acid by a nonreceptor-mediated mechanism.

All receptors have an *endogenous ligand* that, when bound, elicits a physiologic response. Drugs alter the normal physiologic activity at a given receptor to produce a desirable therapeutic effect.

There are several general types of receptor classes (Table 1-1):

- Enzymatic receptors, such as **tyrosine kinase receptors**
- Ion channels, such as **nicotinic cholinergic receptors**
- G protein-coupled receptors, such as **muscarinic cholinergic receptors**
- Cytosolic receptors, such as **nucleic acids**

AGONISTS

An agonist is a receptor activator that produces a physiologic response similar to the effect of the endogenous ligand. The affinity of the drug molecule for the receptor and the intrinsic activity of the drug molecule at the receptor depend on the molecule's structure. The common types of antagonists are:

Full agonist—A drug that can elicit the **maximum** possible response at a receptor

Partial agonist—A drug whose maximal effect at a receptor is **less than** that of other agonists at the same receptor. A partial agonist may appear to be an antagonist in the presence of a full agonist.

ANTAGONISTS

An antagonist is a compound that interferes with the action of an endogenous ligand or an exogenous drug. Antagonists can exert their effects in several ways. Following are the common types of pharmacologic antagonists:

TABLE 1-1	G Protein α-Subunit Classes and Related Receptors, Effectors, and Second Messengers		
G_α CLASS	EXAMPLES OF RECEPTORS	RELATED EFFECTOR	EFFECT ON SECOND MESSENGER SYSTEM
G_s	β-adrenergic, histamine, glucagon, serotonin, vasopressin, other hormones	Adenylyl cyclase	Increases cAMP concentration
$G_{i\,(1,2,3)}$	α-adrenergic, muscarinic acetylcholine, opioids, serotonin	Adenylyl cyclase	Decreases cAMP concentration
G_{olf}	Odorant receptors in olfactory epithelium	Adenylyl cyclase	Increases cAMP concentration
G_o	Acetylcholine receptors in endothelial cells, neurotransmitters in brain	Phospholipase C	Increases IP_3, DAG concentrations
G_q	α_2-adrenergic, bomesin, serotonin (5-HT$_{1C}$)	Phospholipase C	Increases IP_3, DAG concentrations
$G_{t\,(1\,and\,2)}$	Rhodopsin	cGMP phosphodiesterase	Decreases cGMP concentration

HARDCORE

The effect of a pharmacologic antagonist is only observable if there is activity at the receptor.

Receptor or pharmacologic antagonist—A compound that has affinity for a receptor but no intrinsic activity at that receptor. A pharmacologic antagonist competes with a receptor agonist for the **same** receptor binding site, thereby diminishing the effect of the agonist.

Functional or physiologic antagonist—An agonist that, when bound to its receptor, produces an effect opposite to that of another agonist acting at a separate receptor.

Chemical antagonist—A compound that acts as an antagonist by reacting chemically with a drug, thereby inactivating it and preventing its action at a receptor.

Dispositional or pharmacokinetic antagonist—A compound that acts as an antagonist by altering the pharmacokinetic properties of a drug, thereby decreasing the bioavailability of the drug and resulting in a decreased concentration of the drug at its receptor.

Binding at a receptor, whether by an agonist or antagonist, can involve one or more of the following types of chemical interactions. The list of bonds below is arranged from strongest (covalent bonding) to weakest (hydrophobic bonding):

- Covalent bonding
- Ionic bonding
- Hydrogen bonding
- Van der Waals forces
- Hydrophobic interactions

The stronger the interaction, the longer the drug molecule will stay bound. For example, a compound that binds covalently to a receptor will have a much longer duration of action at the receptor than a drug that binds due to van der Waals forces.

Dose-response relationships

The effect observed upon administration of a drug is proportional to the number of receptors that are occupied by the drug. A maximum response is elicited once a certain number of receptors are occupied. In order to achieve a maximal effect, all of the receptors may not need to be stimulated.

$$\text{Observed effect} = (\text{Maximal effect}) \times (\text{fraction of receptors occupied})$$

The fraction of receptors occupied is given by:

$$\frac{[D]}{K_D + [D]}$$

$[D]$ = The concentration of drug at the receptor
K_D = The drug-receptor dissociation constant, which equals K_2/K_1.
K_1 and K_2 = Rate constants from the equation in Figure 1-4.

As the concentration of the drug at the receptor increases, the observed effect will increase until a maximum effect is attained. This relationship can be expressed graphically as a **dose-response curve** (Figure 1-5).

$$\text{Drug} + \text{Receptor} \underset{K1}{\overset{K2}{\rightleftharpoons}} \text{Drug–Receptor Complex} \longrightarrow \text{Effect}$$

Figure 1-4 Drug-receptor dissociation and effect.

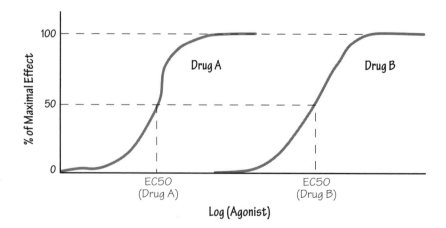

Figure 1-5 Dose-response curves for two different drugs, A and B. Drugs A and B have equal efficacy; however, drug A is more potent than drug B.

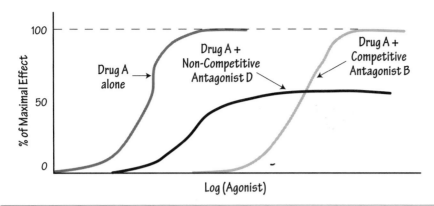

Figure 1-6 Dose response curves for drug A alone, drug A in the presence of a competitive antagonist, B, and drug A in the presence of a noncompetitive antagonist, D. Note that the competitive antagonist is surmountable, whereas the effect of the noncompetitive antagonist cannot be overcome at any dose.

Potency is the power of a drug to produce a desired effect. Quantitatively, potency is *inversely proportional* to the EC_{50} (the concentration of a drug necessary to produce a half-maximal response). In Figure 1-5, drug A is more potent than drug B since it is able to produce the same effect at a lower concentration.

The **maximal efficacy** is the maximum response that a given drug can produce. While drug A is more potent than drug B, drug B is just as efficacious as drug A since it is able to produce the same maximal effect, albeit at a higher dose (see Figure 1-5).

In Figure 1-6, the leftmost curve represents the response to a drug, A, alone. The rightmost curve depicts the response to drug A in the presence of a receptor antagonist, B. In the presence of antagonist B, a greater concentration of drug A is required to produce the same response as drug A alone. Note that eventually, as the concentration of drug A increases, a maximal effect is reached. This type of antagonism is called **competitive** or **surmountable antagonism**.

Now suppose that instead of antagonist B, a different compound, antagonist D, is administered before drug A. The effect of antagonist D on the response to drug A is also depicted in Figure 1-6. Notice that as the concentration of drug A is increased, a maximum effect is achieved, but the efficacy of drug A is reduced. The effect of antagonist D is said to be **insurmountable**. This type of antagonism is called **noncompetitive antagonism**. A noncompetitive antagonist prevents a drug from producing a maximal response at any concentration.

For a pharmacologic antagonist, competitive antagonism indicates that the antagonist binds reversibly, while noncompetitive antagonism indicates that the antagonist is binding irreversibly. If the antagonist is not a pharmacologic antagonist, and therefore binds at a site other than the drug-binding site on the receptor, it cannot be determined if the binding is reversible or irreversible.

Drug-Drug Interactions

Many patients take multiple drugs at the same time. Several terms describe the basic types of interactions that can occur between drugs.

- *Addition*—The combined effect of the drugs is equal to the sum of the individual effects.
- *Synergism*—The combined effect of the drugs is greater than the sum of the individual effects.
- *Potentiation*—An increase in the effect of a drug in the presence of a second drug that has no effect by itself on the system of interest.
- *Antagonism*—A drug interferes with the action of a second drug.

CHAPTER 2

Central Nervous System Pharmacology

The USMLE and shelf exam will test you on a multitude of drug classes that affect the central nervous system (CNS), including *antidepressants, antibipolar agents, antipsychotics, anxiolytics, opiates, antiparkinsonian drugs, anesthetics, migraine medications,* and *antiepileptics.* It can be mentally challenging to sort these drugs because of overlapping mechanisms of action, side effects, and usage, but it is very important to know which drugs are in each class and the general mechanism of action and major side effects for each class. You will find that the shelf and board exams put a high priority on testing these concepts.

ANTIDEPRESSANTS

Tricyclics: *Imipramine, amitriptyline, nortriptyline, desipramine, clomipramine, doxepin*
Monoamine oxidase inhibitors (MAOIs): *Phenelzine, tranylcypromine*
Serotonin-selective reuptake inhibitors (SSRIs): *Sertraline, paroxetine, fluoxetine, italopram, citalopram*
Heterocyclics: *Trazodone, bupropion, venlafaxine, mirtazapine, nefazadone*

Depression is one of the most common psychiatric disorders (lifetime prevalence: 15% to 25%). Patients suffering from this disorder often present clinically with the inability to experience pleasure, fatigue, decreased concentration, guilt, and weight change. Pathophysiologically, the etiology of depression is unclear, although an imbalance in the levels of the amine neurotransmitters **serotonin (5-HT)**, **norepinephrine (NE)**, and **dopamine** in the central nervous system (CNS) may play a role (this is often referred to as the "amine hypothesis"). Many of the antidepressants change levels of neurotransmitters within the neuronal synaptic cleft (at least transiently), and this may contribute to their antidepressant effect. However, the correlation between neurotransmitter levels and depression is unclear, and therefore the exact mechanisms of the antidepressive effects of many of the drugs used to treat depression are unclear.

Tricyclic Antidepressants (TCAs)

Tertiary amine tricyclics: *Amitriptyline, Clomipramine, Imipramine, Doxepin*

- Remember *T-ACID.*

Secondary amine tricyclics: *Amoxapine, Nortriptyline, Desipramine*

- Remember *SAND.*

Indications and Usage—Severe major depression, panic disorder, neuralgia

Mechanism of Action—The exact mechanism of the antidepressant effect of the TCAs is unclear. However, the **inhibition of presynaptic reuptake of norepinephrine and serotonin** appears to be involved, resulting in increased concentrations of these monoamines in the synaptic cleft.

Side Effects—Secondary amine TCAs are more specific for blocking NE and 5-HT reuptake. Thus, while both secondary and tertiary TCAs have side effects, **tertiary TCAs are "dirtier" drugs** (i.e., less specific for NE and 5-HT), and thus tend to be associated with more side effects, such as:

- **α-Adrenergic receptor blockade**: Orthostatic hypotension and reflex tachycardia
- **Muscarinic receptor blockade**: Urinary retention, constipation, blurred vision, dry mouth
- **Histamine receptor blockade**: Sedation

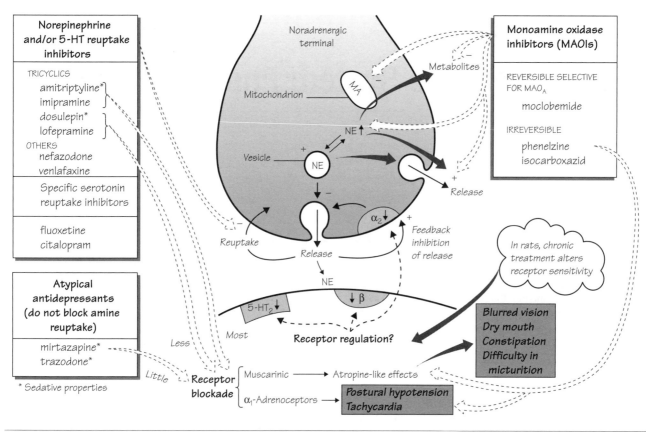

Figure 2-1 **Overview of antidepressants.** (Reprinted with permission from Neal MJ Medical Pharmacology at a Glance. 4th ed. Blackwell Publishing, 2002:62.)

HARDCORE

Clinical improvement in patients taking these drugs typically takes 2–4 weeks.

HARDCORE

MAOIs are usually the *last choice* of antidepressant because of their potentially dangerous side effects.

HARDCORE

Tyramine is commonly found in *cheese and wine*; therefore, patients shouldn't consume cheese, wine, or any food containing tyramine while taking an MAOI.

HARDCORE

Concurrent use of *meperidine* (an opioid agonist) and an MAOI can result in a hypertensive crisis.

HARDCORE

A "washout" period of 2 weeks is recommended when switching from an MAOI to any other antidepressant, because of the long half-life of the MAOIs.

Monoamine Oxidase Inhibitors (MAOIs)

 Nonselective MAOIs: *Phenelzine, tranylcypromine*

Indications and Usage—Atypical depression, anxiety, hypochondriasis

Mechanism of Action—The exact mechanism of the antidepressant effect of the MAOIs is unclear. However, the *inhibition of the enzyme monoamine oxidase (MAO), which metabolizes catecholamine neurotransmitters in the presynaptic nerve terminal*, appears to be involved. Inhibition of MAO results in increased levels of NE and 5-HT within neurons and subsequently in the synaptic cleft.

Side Effects

- *Hypertensive crisis following tyramine ingestion* or with concurrent use of sympathomimetic agents, such as decongestants, stimulants or weight loss aids

- Orthostatic hypotension, weight gain, insomnia

- *Serotonin syndrome if used in conjunction with a serotonin reuptake inhibitor*

Selective-Serotonin Reuptake Inhibitors (SSRIs)

 Sertraline, paroxetine, fluoxetine, citalopram

Indications and Usage—Depression, obsessive-compulsive disorder, premenstrual syndrome, bulimia nervosa, anorexia nervosa

Mechanism of Action—SSRIs inhibit the *presynaptic reuptake of 5-HT* resulting in increased concentrations of 5-HT in the synaptic cleft.

Side Effects—This class is considered first line for depression because these drugs have *fewer side effects than other antidepressants*. The most troublesome side effects include:

- *Diminished libido with delayed ejaculation* (a common reason for noncompliance)

- CNS stimulation including insomnia, tremor, and vomiting

- *Serotonin syndrome*: Hyperpyrexia, muscle rigidity, confusion, cardiovascular collapse, coma, and death. This syndrome is associated with patients taking both SSRIs and MAOIs.

- Withdrawal occurs when SSRIs are discontinued suddenly and includes dizziness, nausea, tremor, anxiety, and dysphoria. Patients should be weaned off of SSRIs slowly.

Heterocyclics

Trazodone, bupropion, venlafaxine, mirtazapine, nefazodone

These drugs are used in the treatment of *major depressive disorders*, but, as with the TCAs and MAOIs, the exact mechanism of their antidepressant effect is unclear. Most of these drugs increase the action of serotonin at its postsynaptic receptor by directly stimulating the postsynaptic 5-HT$_1$ receptors, or by blocking presynpatic 5-HT$_2$ receptors, resulting in inhibition of the negative feedback 5-HT.

VENLAFAXINE

Indications and Usage—Depression and generalized anxiety disorder

Mechanism of Action—Blocks the reuptake of *serotonin*, *dopamine*, and *NE*

Side Effects—*Stimulation*, including anxiety, insomnia, agitation; dose-dependent elevation in diastolic blood pressure

- Venla**f**axine—"Vennie la**f**s when he is anxious" (*for the treatment of anxiety disorder*)

MIRTAZAPINE

Indications and Usage—Depression, especially associated with insomnia or agitation

Mechanism of Action—*Blocks the 5-HT$_2$ receptors*, resulting in inhibition of the negative feedback of serotonin on the presynaptic neuron. This results in an increased release of serotonin from the neuron, increased levels of serotonin in the synapse, and increased 5-HT$_1$-receptor stimulation. *Mirtazapine also blocks α$_2$-adrenergic receptors*, resulting in inhibition of the negative feedback on the presynaptic neuron. This results in an increased release of norepinephrine and serotonin.

Side Effects—Antihistaminic effects leading to *increased appetite and increased sedation*

BUPROPION

Indications and Usage—Smoking cessation and depression

Mechanism of Action—Inhibits reuptake of amine neurotransmitters

Side Effects—Dry mouth, agitation, and aggravation of psychosis

- Bu**pro**pion: "*a pro at smoking cessation.*"

TRAZODONE

Indications and Usage—Depression, especially associated with insomnia

Mechanism of Action—*Inhibits serotonin reuptake*

Side Effects—Sedation, nausea, postural hypotension

NEFAZODONE

Indications and Usage—Depression

Mechanism of Action—Inhibits *norepinephrine* and *serotonin reuptake*, and *antagonizes 5-HT$_2$ receptors*, resulting in increased serotonin levels in the synapse and increased 5-HT$_1$ receptor stimulation

Side Effects—Hepatotoxicity

- "Ne**FAZ**odone won't **FAZe** your sex life!"

MOOD STABILIZERS

Lithium, valproic acid, carbamazepine

Bipolar disorder is a clinical disorder in which depressed patients alternate between periods of mania (episodes of abnormally elevated mood characterized clinically by elevated energy, decreased need to sleep, pressured speech, and increased risk-taking behavior) and periods of depression. Treatment is geared toward stabilizing the patient's mood at an even level and limiting the highs and lows that are associated with this disorder.

LITHIUM

Indications and Usage—Bipolar affective disorder; to prevent acute manic events, depressive episodes, and help limit future relapses (*mood stabilization*)

Mechanism of Action—*The exact mechanism of action of lithium is unclear;* however, alteration of cation transport across nerve cell membranes, inhibition of second messenger systems involving the phosphatidylinositol cycle, or alterations in neurotransmitter release may play a role in its clinical effects.

Side Effects—Tremor, *hypothyroidism*, weight gain, acne

HARDCORE

The SSRI *paroxetine*, an anxiolytic, is paradoxically associated with **increased anxiety** during the first 2 weeks of use.

HARDCORE

Fluoxetine is also commonly used for obsessive-compulsive disorder.

HARDCORE

Fluoxetine has the longest half-life of any of the SSRIs; therefore, the withdrawal syndrome associated with fluoxetine is less severe than with other SSRIs.

HARDCORE

Venlafaxine is particularly useful in depressed patients with anorexia, because it stimulates the appetite.

HARDCORE

Mirtazapine can elevate serum cholesterol.

HARDCORE

The trade name of *mirtazapine* is **Remeron**, or "**R.E.M. Is On**" because of its sedating side effects.

HARDCORE

Bupropion does not cause weight gain, sedation, or sexual dysfunction, because there is no effect on serotonin.

HARDCORE

Priapism can occur in patients taking trazodone.

HARDCORE

Lithium is contraindicated in patients taking thiazide diuretics or metronidazole, or who have alterations in amount of dietary sodium.

HARDCORE

Lithium can act as an **ADH antagonist** resulting in nephrogenic diabetes insipidus.

HARDCORE

Lithium is teratogenic if take during the first trimester of pregnancy.

VALPROIC ACID

Indications and Usage—Bipolar affective disorder; myoclonic and absence seizures

Mechanism of Action—*The exact mechanism of action of valproic acid is unclear.* Enhanced GABA action at inhibitory synapses, prevention of repetitive firing of neurons, and blockade of NMDA receptor-mediated excitation are several possibilities.

Side Effects—Hepatic toxicity, rash, alopecia, fetal spina bifida, and increased bleeding time (due to thrombocytopenia and the inhibition of platelet aggregation)

CARBAMAZEPINE

Indications and Usage—Partial and tonic-clonic seizures; trigeminal neuralgia; manic-depressive disorder

Mechanism of Action—Blockade of sodium channels and inhibition of the generation of repetitive action potentials account for carbamazepine's anticonvulsant activity. Carbamazepine's effect in manic-depressive disorder may be due to either its ability to inhibit norepinephrine reuptake at neurons or its ability to potentiate the action of GABA at postsynaptic neurons.

Side Effects—Hepatic toxicity, agranulocytosis, coma, respiratory depression

ANTIPSYCHOTICS (NEUROLEPTICS)

Typical: *Thioridazine, haloperidol, fluphenazine, chlorpromazine*
Atypical: *Clozapine, olanzapine, risperidone, quetiapine*

Neuroleptics are used clinically to treat schizophrenia, delirium, and mania. These agents act primarily by competitively blocking CNS dopamine receptors, which explains why the most common, and serious, side effects seen with these agents resemble Parkinson's disease, a disease characterized by the loss of nigrostriatal dopaminergic neurons. These unwanted side effects led to the development of the newer "atypical" antipsychotics. Atypical antipsychotics have a higher affinity for serotonin receptors than for dopamine receptors, and therefore have a lower incidence of extrapyramidal side effects.

Typical Antipsychotics

Haloperidol, fluphenazine, thiothixene, chlorpromazine, thioridazine

Indications and Usage—Schizophrenia and psychosis

- Typical antipsychotics are most effective at treating the *positive symptoms of schizophrenia,* including delusions, hallucinations, and disorganized speech or behavior.

Mechanism of Action—*Blockade of dopamine D_2 receptors*

Side Effects

- **Extrapyramidal effects**: Refers to movements that *do not* originate from the pyramidal (corticospinal) tracts and include:
  - **Acute dystonia**—Muscle spasms of tongue, neck, and face
  - **Akathisia**—Motor restlessness, especially of the legs
  - **Parkinsonian symptoms**—Cogwheel rigidity, resting tremors, and abnormal gait
  - **Tardive dyskinesia**—Oral-facial movements (*irreversible*)
- **Blockade of muscarinic, α-adrenergic**, and **histamine receptors**: Results in antimuscarinic effects, hypotension, and sedation, respectively
- **Neuroleptic malignant syndrome (NMS)**: Includes muscular rigidity, hyperpyrexia, and altered mental status.
- Treat patients with NMS with *dantrolene* (blocks calcium channels) and dopamine agonists (*bromocriptine*).

Atypical Antipsychotics

CROQ: Clozapine, Risperidone, Olanzapine, Quetiapine

Indications and Usage—Used for *both the positive and negative (flat affect) symptoms* of schizophrenia

Mechanism of Action—These drugs *block both dopamine receptors and 5-HT$_2$ receptors*.

Side Effects—Weight gain; extrapyramidal and anticholinergic effects. Because these drugs do not act solely on dopamine receptors, *side effects are milder than the typical antipsychotics*.

ANXIOLYTICS

Benzodiazepines: *Diazepam, lorazepam, midazolam, chlordiazepoxide, triazolam, oxazepam*

Barbiturates: *Phenobarbital, pentobarbital, thiopental, secobarbital*

Azaspirones: *Buspirone*

Anxiety is an abnormal and overwhelming sense of apprehension or fear that may be accompanied by physiological signs. These signs include increased autonomic activity (sweating, tachycardia) and motor tension. Anxiety may occur due to a person's environment (situational anxiety) or secondary to another medical condition, such as angina, which may require additional treatment.

Benzodiazepines: The "-am" drugs

Diazepam, lorazepam, midazolam, chlordiazepoxide, triazolam, oxazepam

Indications and Usage—Anxiety, spasticity (*diazepam*), and detoxification/alcohol withdrawal

Mechanism of Action—These agents promote GABA-mediated inhibitory effects in the CNS by *increasing the frequency of chloride channel opening*.

- The short-acting benzodiazepines Lorazepam, Oxazepam, and Triazolam *don't act for a LOT of time*

Side Effects—Benzodiazepine use can cause CNS depression and dependence. The most common side effects are sedation, ataxia, anterograde amnesia, and behavioral disinhibition.

Barbiturates: The "-tal" drugs

Phenobarbital, pentobarbital, thiopental, secobarbital

Indications and Usage—Anxiety, seizures, insomnia

Mechanism of Action—These agents promote GABA-mediated CNS inhibitory effects by *increasing the duration of chloride channel opening*.

Side Effects—CNS depression with respiratory failure; dependence

Azaspirones: The "-spirone" drugs

Buspirone

Indication and Usage—Generalized anxiety

Mechanism of Action—The exact mechanism of buspirone's anxiolytic effect is unknown, but stimulation of *5-HT$_{1A}$ receptors or dopamine D$_2$ receptors* may be involved.

Side Effects—Headache, dizziness, and nausea

OPIOID ANALGESICS

Full agonists: *Morphine, meperidine, fentanyl, methadone, heroin, hydromorphone*

Partial agonists: *Codeine, hydrocodone, oxycodone, propoxyphene*

Mixed agonist and antagonist: *Pentazocine, nalbuphine, butorphanol*

There are four types of endogenous opioid receptors, but the most important clinically is the *mu opioid receptor*. The mu opioid receptor mediates the analgesic effects of opioids, either endogenous enkephalins or exogenously administered opioids. Activation of sigma and mu opioid receptors is responsible for the undesirable effects of opioids, including euphoria, respiratory depression, and dependence.

Full and Partial Agonists

Morphine, meperidine, fentanyl, methadone, heroin, hydromorphone, codeine, hydrocodone, oxycodone, propoxyphene

Indications and Usage—Relief of pain; *methadone* is used to treat heroin addiction

Mechanism of Action—*Stimulate opioid receptors*

Side Effects—Opioids are highly addictive and can also cause CNS and respiratory depression; miosis, constipation, euphoria, and hallucinations may also occur.

Mixed Agonists/Antagonists

Pentazocine, nalbuphine, butorphanol

HARDCORE

Diazepam is indicated for status epilepticus.

HARDCORE

Benzodiazepines and barbiturates both act on GABA receptors, but benzodiazepines increase the **frequency** of chloride channel opening, whereas barbiturates increase the **duration** of channel opening.

HARDCORE

Flumazenil acts as a competitive antagonist to GABA receptors and can be used as an antidote for benzodiazepine overdose.

HARDCORE

An overdose of benzodiazepines alone does not cause fatal respiratory depression. However, if used in combination with alcohol and barbiturates, the CNS depressant effects are potentiated and respiratory depression may occur.

HARDCORE

Thiopental is used for the induction of anesthesia.

HARDCORE

These drugs induce the cytochrome P450 enzyme.
- **BAR**biturates raise the **BAR** for P450 metabolism.

HARDCORE

Barbiturates are contraindicated in patients with porphyria.

HARDCORE

Unlike the benzodiazepines and barbiturates, buspirone does not have any hypnotic or anticonvulsant properties, and does not cause dependence.

HARDCORE

Fentanyl is 80 times more potent than *morphine*.

HARDCORE

Meperidine antagonizes muscarinic acetylcholine receptors. Therefore, instead of causing pupil constriction, *meperidine* causes pupil dilation.

HARDCORE

Naloxone and *naltrexone* are opioid antagonists and are used to block or reverse the effects of opioids in an overdose situation.

HARDCORE

Tolerance is a common problem for patients using opioids chronically:
- Patients never become tolerant to the miotic and constipating effects of opioid agonists.
- Use of an opioid will cause cross-tolerance to other opioids.

HARDCORE

Mixed agonists-antagonists are less likely to cause dependence than full agonists.

HARDCORE

Pentazocine should not be used by patients who have angina, because it can increase the work of the heart by increasing the aortic and pulmonary arterial pressures. Pentazocine also decreases renal plasma flow.

HARDCORE

Mixed agonist-antagonists such as *pentazocine* should not be used with opioid agonists such as morphine because a partial antagonist can precipitate an opioid withdrawal syndrome.

HARDCORE

Levodopa is used for Parkinson's disease because it crosses the blood-brain barrier, whereas dopamine cannot.

HARDCORE

Levodopa is given clinically with the peripheral decarboxylase inhibitor *carbidopa*. *Carbidopa* prevents the peripheral conversion of *levodopa* to dopamine and does not cross the blood-brain barrier. Thus, this drug combination allows for increased dopamine production within the CNS, but also limits peripheral dopamine production and its associated side effects.

HARDCORE

Levodopa has an extremely short half-life.

The "**on-off effect**" is the unpredictable fluctuation between mobility and immobility that can occur in Parkinson's patients following a drop in plasma levodopa levels.

Indication and Usage—Analgesia

Mechanism of Action—Agonist at kappa and/or delta opioid receptors and antagonist at mu receptors

Side Effects—Constipation, respiratory depression, increases in blood pressure, hallucinations, nightmares

DRUGS USED TO TREAT PARKINSON'S DISEASE

> **Agents that act to increase dopamine levels:** *Selegiline, levodopa/carbidopa, bromocriptine, amantadine*
>
> **Muscarinic antagonists:** *Trihexyphenidyl, benztropine*

Normally, dopaminergic neurons located in the substantia nigra oppose the effect of cholinergic neurons in the corpus striatum the GABAergic neurons in the corpus striatum (Figure 2-2). In Parkinson's disease, the dopaminergic neurons originating in the substantia nigra are lost over time, resulting in an *imbalance between the cholinergic pathway and the dopaminergic pathway* and the symptoms of Parkinson's disease.

The treatment of Parkinson's disease focuses on two processes:

1. *Increasing* the amount of dopamine and its duration of action in the brain
2. *Inhibiting* the cholinergic pathway by blocking muscarinic receptors in the brain

Agents That Act to Increase Dopamine Levels

LEVODOPA (L-DOPA)

Mechanism of Action—A *precursor of dopamine* that is converted to dopamine, both in the CNS and peripherally

Side Effects—Arrhythmias, anorexia, nausea, and postural hypotension can occur if levodopa is converted to dopamine in the peripheral vascular system (use *carbidopa* to prevent this). Dyskinesias, vivid dreams, hallucinations, and confusion can occur from excess dopamine production in the CNS.

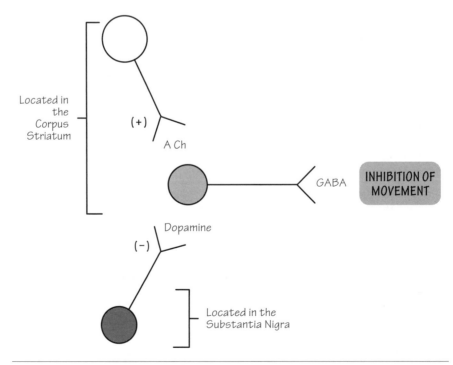

Figure 2-2 Schematic of the nigrostriatal pathway. Normally, firing of dopaminergic neurons located in the substantia nigra results in inhibition of GABAergic neurons in the corpus striatum, resulting in disinhibition of movement. Firing of cholinergic neurons in the corpus striatum stimulates GABA-mediated inhibition of movement. In Parkinson's disease, the dopaminergic neurons originating in the substantia nigra are lost over time, resulting in unopposed cholinergic stimulation of the GABAergic neurons in the corpus striatum, and the inhibition of movement.

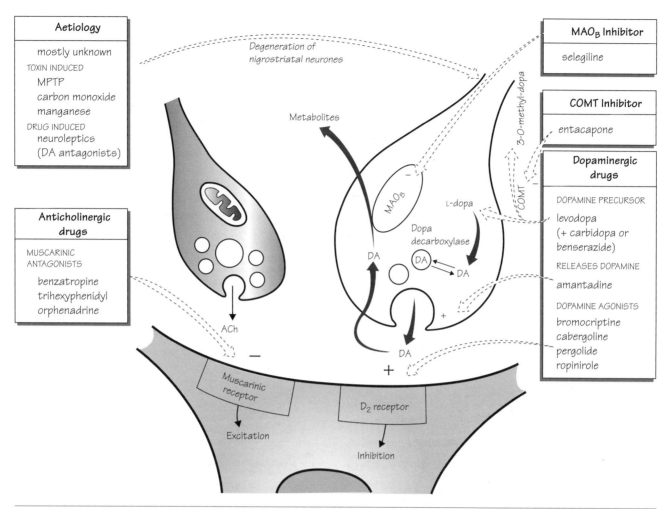

Figure 2-3 Drugs used to treat Parkinson's disease. (Reprinted with permission from Neal MJ. Medical Pharmacology at a Glance. 4th ed. Oxford: Blackwell Publishing, 2002:58.)

SELEGILINE

Mechanism of Action—Selectively *inhibits MAO-B*, thereby decreasing the metabolism of dopamine and prolonging its action. Since levodopa is converted to dopamine, concurrent use of selegiline prolongs the effect of levodopa and may allow a reduction in the dose of levodopa that is needed.

Side Effects—Orthostatic hypotension, weight gain, insomnia

BROMOCRIPTINE

Mechanism of action—A partial dopamine agonist

Side effects

- **Peripheral**: Cardiac arrhythmias, postural hypotension, worsening of existing peptic ulcers
- **Central**: Hallucinations

AMANTADINE

Indications and Usage—Primarily an antiviral drug used to treat influenza that is also used in Parkinson's disease and in conjunction with antipsychotics

Mechanism of Action—Increases dopamine release

Side Effects—Tolerance; antimuscarinic effects, including orthostatic hypotension, urinary retention, and dry mouth

Muscarinic Antagonists

 Benztropine, trihexyphenidyl

Mechanism of Action—Antagonize muscarinic cholinergic receptors

Side Effects—Typical antimuscarinic effects, including dry mouth, pupillary dilation, constipation, urinary retention

HARDCORE

Recall that inhibition of MAO results in increased levels of dopamine, NE, and 5-HT within neurons and subsequently in the synaptic cleft, and that there are two subtypes of MAO: *MAO-A*, which preferentially oxidizes serotonin and norepinephrine, and *MAO-B*, which is located centrally and preferentially oxidizes dopamine. Most MAOIs react nonspecifically with both MAO-A and MAO-B. However, *selegiline* selectively inhibits only MAO-B, resulting in fewer drug interactions and a lower risk of hypertension with tyramine-rich foods.

ANESTHETICS

There are *four stages of anesthesia*, all of which are characterized by an increasing CNS depression:

1. **Analgesia**—Characterized by reduced awareness of pain, but no loss of consciousness
2. **Excitement**—Characterized by delirium and violent behavior with a rise in blood pressure
   - This stage is avoided by administering a short-acting barbiturate before the inhaled anesthetic.
3. **Surgical anesthesia**—Characterized by relaxation of skeletal muscle and loss of sensory and autonomic reflexes, but maintenance of regular respiration
4. **Medullary paralysis**—Characterized by depression of the respiratory center, which can possibly be fatal; typically seen with too much anesthetic and obviously *not desirable*

The potency of inhaled anesthetics is determined by the *minimum alveolar concentration (MAC)*, which represents the concentration of gas needed to eliminate movement in 50% of patients.

- Potent anesthetics have a <u>small MAC</u>: *Halothane (lowest MAC) > isoflurane > enflurane (highest MAC)*
- Less potent anesthetics have a <u>large MAC</u>: *Nitrous oxide*

An anesthetic's solubility in the blood is determined by the drug's *blood/gas partition coefficient*.

- Drugs with <u>low solubility</u> do not easily dissolve in blood and therefore reach steady state quickly, causing rapid induction and rapid recovery (e.g., *nitrous oxide*).
- Drugs with <u>high solubility</u> in blood reach steady state more slowly, causing slower induction and recovery (e.g., *halothane*).

The anesthetic agents can be divided into three categories:

1. Inhaled anesthetics
2. Intravenous anesthetics
3. Local anesthetics

Inhaled Anesthetics: The "*-ane*" drugs

 Halothane, enflurane, isoflurane, sevoflurane, nitrous oxide

Mechanism of Action—These drugs interact with GABA and other central neurotransmitter receptors, resulting in a decrease in spontaneous and evoked activity of central neurons.

Side Effects—Increased cerebral blood flow, respiratory and myocardial depression, nausea and vomiting. Agent-specific effects include:

- *Halothane*: Hepatotoxicity and arrhythmias
- *Enflurane*: Proconvulsant and some hepatotoxicity risk
- *Isoflurane*: Initially stimulates respiratory reflexes
- *Nitrous oxide*: Diffusion hypoxia, no muscle relaxation

Intravenous Anesthetics

 Thiopental, propofol, midazolam, ketamine, morphine, fentanyl

Intravenous anesthetics have a much more rapid onset of action than inhaled anesthetics, and are therefore commonly used for induction of anesthesia. Intravenous anesthetics are also used as the sole anesthetic in short surgical procedures.

THIOPENTAL

Indications and Usage—Rapid induction of anesthesia in short procedures

Side Effects—Decreases cerebral blood flow

PROPOFOL

Indications and Usage—Commonly used for *rapid induction*

Side Effects—Reduces intracranial pressure

MIDAZOLAM

Indications and Usage—Endoscopic procedures and in combination with gaseous anesthetics

Side Effects—*Amnesia*, post-op respiratory depression

KETAMINE

Indications and Usage—Pediatrics ("**ket** for **kids**"), a *dissociative anesthetic*

Side Effects—Hallucinations, PCP analog ("*special K*"—like PCP)

HARDCORE

Inhaled anesthetics can cause *malignant hyperthermia* (long periods of sustained muscle contractions and with an accompanying rise in body temperature) on rare occasions. Malignant hyperthermia can be treated with the calcium channel blocker *dantrolene*.

Morphine/Fentanyl

Indications and Usage—General anesthesia, pain control

Side effects—Respiratory depression

Local Anesthetics

 Esters—One "I" in the name: *Procaine, cocaine, tetracaine*
Amides—Two "I"'s in the name: *LIdocaine, bupIvacaine*

These agents are used to prevent pain by causing a reversible block of conduction along nerve fibers. Local anesthetics act *within the neuron to block sodium channels*, preventing the generation of action potentials. The local anesthetics can be classified according to the type of linkage they contain, either an ester or amide linkage. Drugs with an ester linkage are metabolized by the esterases in the blood, whereas those with an amide linkage are metabolized by hepatic enzymes. Some patients will develop an allergic reaction to one type of local anesthetic. Know how to pick which type of local anesthetic that will *not result in an allergic complication* (i.e., if the patient is allergic to an ester choose an amide and vice versa).

Indications and Usage—Analgesia during minor surgical procedures; spinal anesthesia

Mechanism of Action—These drugs block sensation by binding to *voltage-gated sodium channels, thereby preventing conduction of nerve action potentials*.

Side Effects—CNS excitation and various cardiovascular effects, including hypertension and cardiac arrhythmias

MUSCLE RELAXANTS

 Baclofen, dantrolene, succinylcholine, tubocurarine, pancuronium, doxacurium

These agents are used to relax skeletal muscle during surgical procedures and to control spastic tone seen in spinal cord patients, multiple sclerosis, and malignant hyperthermia. Muscle relaxants may act centrally (e.g., *baclofen*), intracellularly (e.g., *dantrolene*), or at the neuromuscular junction as either competitive antagonists of nicotinic acetylcholine receptors (e.g., *tubocurarine*) or depolarizing blockers (e.g., *succinylcholine*). *Competitive antagonists* compete with acetylcholine for nicotinic receptors at the neuromuscular endplate, blocking muscular contraction. *Depolarizing agents* act by first triggering the opening of ion channels and depolarization; however, because the drug slowly dissociates from receptors, a prolonged depolarization occurs and blocks subsequent depolarizing stimuli and the associated muscular contraction.

Baclofen

Indications and Usage—*Reversible spasticity* associated with multiple sclerosis or spinal cord lesions

Mechanism of Action—*Inhibits* the transmission of reflexes at the level of the spinal cord, probably by *GABA-mediated hyperpolarization* of primary afferent fiber terminals

Side Effects—Drowsiness, weakness, dizziness

Dantrolene

Indications and Usage—Malignant hyperthermia

Mechanism of Action—Binds to the ryanodine receptor and *interferes with the release of calcium from the sarcoplasmic reticulum* in skeletal muscle, thereby preventing the increase in intracellular calcium normally associated with skeletal muscle contraction

Side Effects—Drowsiness, dizziness, pericarditis

Tubocurarine, Pancuronium, Doxacurium

Indications and Usage—Muscular relaxation during surgical procedures

Mechanism of Action—Competitive antagonist at the nicotinic acetylcholine receptor (*nondepolarizing muscle relaxant*)

Side Effects—Hypotension, histamine release

Succinylcholine

Indications and Usage—Muscular relaxation during surgical procedures

Mechanism of Action—Produces prolonged depolarization of skeletal muscle, which prevents subsequent depolarizing stimuli from causing muscular contraction (*depolarizing muscle relaxant*)

Side Effects—Postoperative muscle pain, hyperkalemia

HARDCORE

These drugs are usually administered with *epinephrine* to produce local vasoconstriction. Local vasoconstriction minimizes the removal of anesthetic from the site of administration by blood flow, resulting in a longer duration of action. However, never use *epinephrine* in fingers, toes, or the penis due to risk of ischemia and death of tissue.

HARDCORE

The order of sensation loss:
1) Pain
2) Temperature
3) Touch
4) Pressure

HARDCORE

Malignant hyperthermia is a rare condition that can be triggered by various stimuli. In response to one of these stimuli, a sudden and protracted release of intracellular calcium stores results in muscle contraction, lactic acid production, and hyperthermia.

HARDCORE

Unlike the nondepolarizing muscle relaxants, the actions of succinylcholine are *not reversed by anticholinesterases*.

DRUGS USED TO TREAT MIGRAINES

5-HT₁ receptor agonists ("-triptans"): *Sumatriptan, zolmitriptan, naratriptan*
Ergot alkaloids: *Ergotamine, dihydroergotamine*
Prophylactic agents: *Methysergide*

The etiology of migraine headaches is currently thought to be associated with the release of vasoactive neuropeptides and the subsequent vasodilation of cranial blood vessels produced by these peptides. The increased blood flow associated with this vasodilation results in leakage of plasma and plasma proteins into the extracellular space, producing edema. The mechanical pressure caused by the edema may be involved in the stimulation of pain receptors in the dura. The cranial blood vessels and the neurons innnervating them contain serotonin receptors (5-HT₁) that, when activated, result in vasoconstriction and inhibition of release of vasodilating neuropeptides, respectively. Treatment of migraines targets these serotonin receptors within the cranial vasculature.

5-HT₁ Receptor Agonists ("-triptans")

Sumatriptan, zolmitriptan, naratriptan

Mechanism of Action—Selective agonist at 5-HT₁ receptors on cranial blood vessels and the neurons innervating them. Stimulation of these receptors results in vasoconstriction and a reduction in the edema and inflammation associated with antidromic neuronal transmission.

Side Effects—**Chest pain** (tightness or pressure in the chest) secondary to drug-induced coronary vasoconstriction; tingling; flushing

ERGOT ALKALOIDS

Ergotamine, dihydroergotamine

Mechanism of Action—**Nonspecific 5-HT agonists**. Stimulation of these receptors results in vasoconstriction and a reduction in the edema and inflammation associated with antidromic neuronal transmission.

Side Effects—These agents are also **contraindicated** in patients with coronary artery disease, angina, or other vascular diseases due to the vasospastic effects of the ergot alkaloids; diarrhea; nausea and vomiting; rebound headaches

Prophylactic Agents

Methysergide

Mechanism of Action—The mechanism of methysergide's prophylactic effect is unknown.

Side Effects—Occur in about 40% of individuals taking methysergide, and include subendocardial fibrosis

ANTIEPILEPTICS

For the most part, the board exam will test you on the classic antiepileptic agents:

Phenytoin, phenobarbital, carbamazepine, ethosuximide, valproic acid

Epilepsy is a chronic disorder characterized by unpredictable, recurrent seizures (abnormal discharge of central neurons resulting in dysfunction of the brain). However, many of the drugs used in the treatment of epilepsy have the same general mechanism of action: *blockade of the electric discharge from a focal area and prevention of the spread of the abnormal electrical discharge to adjacent brain areas.*

Based on electroencephalographic data, several different types of epilepsy exist.

Partial/Focal Epilepsy

These seizures are focal, have a localized neurologic symptom that can be sensory, motor, or psychomotor, and involve only one cerebral hemisphere. Although partial seizures can be divided into simple and complex, both simple and complex seizures are treated using the same medications.

Treatment

Primarily phenytoin, carbamazepine, also primidone, lamotrigine, gabapentin, topiramate

---

HARDCORE

These drugs should be taken at the onset of migraine symptoms.

HARDCORE

These drugs are *contraindicated* in patients with coronary artery disease, angina, or other vascular diseases, because of the vasospastic effects the "triptans."

HARDCORE

Caffeine increases the effectiveness of the ergot alkaloids.

HARDCORE

The ergot alkaloids are typically given in combination with an antiemetic such as prochlorperazine.

HARDCORE

Dihydroergotamine has fewer side effects than ergotamine and does not produce rebound headaches.

HARDCORE

Methysergide is an ergot alkaloid derivative, but it does not possess the vasospastic activity associated with other ergot alkaloids.

HARDCORE

Patients **DO NOT** lose consciousness with a simple partial seizure, whereas patients with complex partial seizures will lose consciousness and will have a postictal period (i.e., a period of disorientation).

Generalized Epilepsy

These seizures involve abnormal electrical discharge throughout both hemispheres of the brain and an immediate loss of consciousness. These seizures can be divided into tonic-clonic, absence, myoclonic, febrile, and status epilepticus types.

Treatment

Tonic-clonic: *Primarily phenytoin and carbamazepine,* **also primidone, lamotrigine, gabapentin, valproic acid, phenobarbital** (*T-C is P-C*)

Absence: *Ethosuximide,* <u>*val*</u>*proic acid,* **clonazepam**

- **It "sux" for "Val" to "absence" from her Step 1 test**

Myoclonic: *Valproic acid,* **clonazepam**

Febrile: *Phenobarbital,* **primidone**

Status epilepticus: *Diazepam, phenytoin,* **phenobarbital**

Drugs Used to Treat Epilepsy

Phenytoin, carbamazepine, phenobarbital, ethosuximide, valproic acid

PHENYTOIN

Indications and Usage—Partial seizures, tonic-clonic seizures, and status epilepticus

Mechanism of Action—Phenytoin alters conductance of major cations (Na^+, K^+, Ca^{2+}) and release of neurotransmitters, and inhibits repetitive firing of neuronal action potentials.

Side Effects—Nystagmus, ataxia, ***gingival hyperplasia***, hirsutism

CARBAMAZEPINE

Indications and Usage—Partial and tonic-clonic seizures

Mechanism of Action—Blockade of sodium channels and inhibition of the generation of repetitive action potentials account for carbamazepine's anticonvulsant activity.

Side Effects—Dose-related rash, transient diplopia, ataxia

PHENOBARBITAL: *The classic antiepileptic*

Indications and Usage—Febrile seizures, tonic-clonic seizures, and status epilepticus

Mechanism of Action—The exact mechanism by which phenobarbital relieves seizures is unknown, but it likely involves promotion of GABA-mediated inhibitory processes.

Side Effects—Sedation, nystagmus, psychosis, Stevens-Johnson syndrome (a disorder characterized by severe erythema multiforme-like eruption of the skin and lesions of the oral, genital, and anal mucosa, including hemorrhagic crusting on the lips and associated fever, headache, and arthralgia)

ETHOSUXIMIDE

Indications and Usage—Absence seizures

Mechanism of Action—Inhibition of T-type Ca^{2+} channels in thalamic neurons involved in absence seizures

Side Effects—Stevens-Johnson syndrome, gastrointestinal discomfort

VALPROIC ACID

Indications and Usage—Myoclonic (DOC) and absence seizures, bipolar disorder

Mechanism of Action—*The exact mechanism of action of valproic acid is unclear.* Enhanced GABA action at inhibitory synapses, prevention of repetitive firing of neurons, and blockade of NMDA receptor-mediated excitation are possibilities.

Side Effects—Nausea, vomiting, and gastrointestinal discomfort are most common.

HARDCORE

Phenytoin interferes with the metabolism of vitamin B_{12} and may cause peripheral neuropathy and megaloblastic anemia.

HARDCORE

Do not give *carbamazepine* for absence or myoclonic seizures.

HARDCORE

Carbamazepine is the drug of choice for the treatment of trigeminal neuralgia.

HARDCORE REVIEW – CNS PHARMACOLOGY

TABLE 2-1   Antidepressants

Drug Class	Drugs	Mechanism of Action	Major Side Effects
Tricyclics	Imipramine, amitriptyline, nortriptyline, desipramine, clomipramine, doxepin	Inhibits the reuptake of norepinephrine and serotonin	Antimuscarinic/anticholinergic, anti-α-adrenergic, and antihistaminic
Monoamine oxidase inhibitors	Phenelzine, tranylcypromine	Inhibits monoamine oxidase enzyme	Hypertensive crisis, serotonin syndrome
Serotonin-selective reuptake inhibitors	Sertraline, paroxetine, fluoxetine, italopram, citalopram	Inhibits reuptake of serotonin	Serotonin syndrome, decreased libido, weight change
Heterocyclics	Venlafaxine	Reuptake blocker of serotonin, dopamine, and NE	Anxiety, insomnia, agitation
	Mirtazapine	Blocks 5-HT$_2$ and α_2 receptors	Antihistamine—increased sedation and appetite
	Bupropion	Reuptake blocker of norepinephrine and dopamine	Agitation, psychosis
	Trazodone	Reuptake blocker of serotonin primarily	Sedation, postural hypotension
	Nefazodone	Reuptake blocker of norepinephrine and serotonin, blocks 5-HT$_2$ receptors	Liver toxicity

TABLE 2-2   Mood Stabilizers

Drug Class	Drugs	Mechanism of Action	Major Side Effects
Lithium	Lithium	Inhibition of the phosphatidylinositol cascade	Tremor, hypothyroidism, weight gain
Valproic acid	Valproic acid	Enhances GABA action at inhibitory synapses	Hepatic toxicity, alopecia, fetal spina bifida
Carbamazepine	Carbamazepine	Blocks sodium channels	Hepatic toxicity, agranulocytosis

TABLE 2-3   Antipsychotics

Drug Class	Drugs	Mechanism of Action	Major Side Effects
Typical	Thioridazine, haloperidol, fluphenazine, chlorpromazine	Blocks D$_2$ receptors	EPS, NMS
Atypical	Clozapine, olanzapine, risperidone, quetiapine	Blocks both dopamine receptors and 5-HT$_2$ receptors	Weight gain, EPS (limited), anticholinergic

TABLE 2-4 Anxiolytics

Drug Class	Drugs	Mechanism of Action	Major Side Effects
Benzodiazepines	Diazepam, Lorazepam, Midazolam, Chlordiazepoxide, Triazolam, Oxazepam	GABA-mediated inhibitory effects by increasing the **frequency** of chloride channel opening	CNS depression and dependence
Barbiturates	Phenobarbital, pentobarbital, thiopental, secobarbital	GABA-mediated inhibitory effects by increasing the **duration** of chloride channel opening	CNS depression with respiratory failure and dependence
Azaspirones	Buspirone	Partial agonists at 5-HT$_{1a}$ receptors	Headache, dizziness, nausea
Benzodiazepine antagonist	Flumazenil	Competitive antagonist at GABA receptors	Can induce withdrawal symptoms

TABLE 2-5 Opioid Analgesics

Drug Class	Drugs	Mechanism of Action	Major Side Effects
Full agonists	Morphine, meperidine, fentanyl, methadone, heroin, hydromorphone	Agonists at endogenous opioid receptors	CNS and respiratory depression
Partial agonists	Codeine, hydrocodone, oxycodone, propoxyphene	Partial agonists at endogenous opioid receptors	CNS and respiratory depression
Mixed agonists and antagonists	Pentazocine, nalbuphine, butorphanol	Agonist at kappa and/or delta receptors and antagonist at mu receptors	Constipation, respiratory depression, hallucinations
Opioid antagonists	Naloxone, naltrexone	Bind opioid receptors but do not elicit a response	Induce withdrawal

TABLE 2-6 Antiparkinsonian drugs

Drug Class	Drugs	Mechanism of Action	Major Side Effects
Drugs that increase dopamine levels	Selegiline	Inhibits MAO-B	Orthostasis, weight gain, insomnia
	Levodopa/carbidopa	Precursor of dopamine; peripheral decarboxylase inhibitor	Arrhythmias, anorexia, CNS stimulation
	Bromocriptine	Partial dopamine agonist	Cardiac arrhythmias, hallucinations
	Amantadine	Increases dopamine release	Anticholinergic
Muscarinic antagonists	Benztropine, trihexyphenidyl	Antagonist at muscarinic cholinergic receptors	Anticholinergic

TABLE 2-7 Anesthetics

Drug Class	Drugs	Mechanism of Action	Major Side Effects
Inhaled anesthetics	Halothane, enflurane, isoflurane, sevoflurane, methoxyflurane, nitrous oxide	Alters the function of GABA, glutamate, and other central receptors	Respiratory and myocardial depression
Intravenous anesthetics	Thiopental	Alters the function of GABA, glutamate, and other central receptors	Decreases cerebral blood flow
	Propofol		Reduces intracranial pressure
	Midazolam		Amnesia, post-op respiratory depression
	Ketamine		Hallucinations
	Morphine/fentanyl		Respiratory depression
Local anesthetics Esters	Procaine, cocaine, tetracaine	Blocks sodium channels	CNS excitation, cardiovascular toxicity
Amides	Lidocaine, bupivacaine	Blocks sodium channels	CNS excitation, cardiovascular toxicity

TABLE 2-8	Muscle Relaxants		
DRUG CLASS	DRUGS	MECHANISM OF ACTION	MAJOR SIDE EFFECTS
Muscle relaxants	Baclofen	Inhibits reflexes in the spinal cord, probably GABA mediated	Weakness, drowsiness
	Dantrolene	Interferes with SR calcium release	Drowsiness, pericarditis
Neuromuscular blockers	Succinylcholine	Blocks the neuromuscular junction *after initial depolarization*	Postoperative muscle pain, hyperkalemia
	Tubocurarine	Blocks the neuromuscular junction with *NO* initial depolarization	Hypotension, histamine release
	Pancuronium	Blocks the neuromuscular junction with *NO* initial depolarization	Hypotension, histamine release
	Doxacurium	Blocks the neuromuscular junction with *NO* initial depolarization	Hypotension, histamine release

TABLE 2-9	Drugs Used to Treat Migraine Headaches		
DRUG CLASS	DRUGS	MECHANISM OF ACTION	MAJOR SIDE EFFECTS
5-HT$_1$ receptor agonists: The triptans	Sumatriptan, zolmitriptan, naratriptan	5-HT$_1$ serotonin receptor agonist, vasoconstriction	Chest pain
Ergot alkaloids	Ergotamine dihydroergotamine	Nonspecific 5-HT agonist, vasoconstriction	Rebound headaches

TABLE 2-10	Hardcore Antiepileptics		
TYPES OF SEIZURES	DRUGS USED FOR TREATMENT	MECHANISM OF ACTION	MAJOR SIDE EFFECTS
Partial, tonic-clonic, and status epilepticus	Phenytoin	Decreases influx of sodium ions	Nystagmus, gingival hyperplasia, hirsutism
Partial and tonic-clonic	Carbamazepine	Decreases sodium-channel activation	Agranulocytosis, aplastic anemia
Febrile, tonic-clonic, and status epilepticus	Phenobarbital	GABA-mediated CNS inhibition by increasing **duration** of chloride channel opening	CNS and respiratory depression
Absence	Ethosuximide	Inhibits T-type calcium channels	Stevens-Johnson syndrome, GI discomfort
Myoclonic and absence	Valproic acid	Decreases sodium-channel activation	Thrombocytopenia, fetal spina bifida

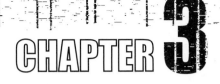

CHAPTER 3

Autonomic Nervous System Pharmacology

The autonomic nervous system is a division of the peripheral nervous system that controls the involuntary responses of the body, such as blood pressure, heart rate, gastrointestinal motility, and pupil diameter. The organization of the autonomic nervous system is based on reflex arcs. Visceral impulses travel via afferent peripheral pathways to the central nervous system, where they are integrated and processed. Efferent pathways then transmit the processed signal to visceral effectors. These visceral effectors include smooth muscle, cardiac muscle, and glands.

The autonomic nervous system is subdivided into two branches, the *parasympathetic nervous system* and the *sympathetic nervous system*. Characteristics of the sympathetic and parasympathetic branches are given in Table 3-1 and are shown in Figure 3-1.

A good way to remember the differences between the sympathetic and parasympathetic nervous system is to think about how your body reacts when *(1) you are attacked by a bear*, or *(2) when you are sitting on the couch*. The *sympathetic nervous system* is responsible for adjusting your body to stressful situation. Therefore, the sympathetic nervous system would be activated in the stressful situations of a bear attack. Visualize what physiologic changes your body would undergo in this situation. Your heart rate and cardiac output would increase, your bronchioles would dilate to increase oxygen supply and uptake, your blood would be shunted from the skin and visceral organs to skeletal muscle to help with running or fighting, your pupils would dilate to increase light intake and improve night and far vision, your urethral sphincter would constrict and intestinal motility would diminish to prevent needless elimination (obviously quite unnecessary while being chased by a bear).

In contrast, the *parasympathetic nervous system* is dominant while you are sitting on your couch watching TV. The parasympathetic nervous system is dominant at rest, and favors increased intestinal motility, relaxation of urethral sphincter tone, increased salivation, constriction of the pupils, decreased heart rate and cardiac output, and bronchoconstriction in the lungs. The increased lung capacity, heart rate, and skeletal muscle blood flow produced in response to sympathetic nervous system activation are not necessary while sitting on the couch. Therefore, the sympathetic nervous system is not as active in this situation.

Therapeutically, the autonomic system can be manipulated to cause a wide variety of physiologic changes. Drugs acting on the autonomic nervous system do so by mimicking or altering the release of endogenous neurotransmitters, as well as by interacting with endogenous receptors. It is, therefore, important to be familiar with each of the endogenous neurotransmitters in the autonomic nervous system and the receptor(s) they act on (Figure 3-2).

TABLE 3-1 General Characteristics of the Autonomic Nervous System

	PARASYMPATHETIC NERVOUS SYSTEM	SYMPATHETIC NERVOUS SYSTEM
Vertebral level of origin	Cervical and sacral	Thoracic and lumbar
Location of ganglia	Near or in target tissue / organ	Close to the spinal column
Ganglionic neurotransmitter	Acetylcholine	Acetylcholine
Ganglionic receptor	Nicotinic	Nicotinic
Preganglionic neuron length	Long	Short
Postganglionic neuron length	Short	Long
Postganglionic terminal neurotransmitter (at target tissue)	Acetylcholine	Norepinephrine
Postganglionic terminal receptor(s) (at target tissue)	Muscarinic	α- and β-Adrenergic

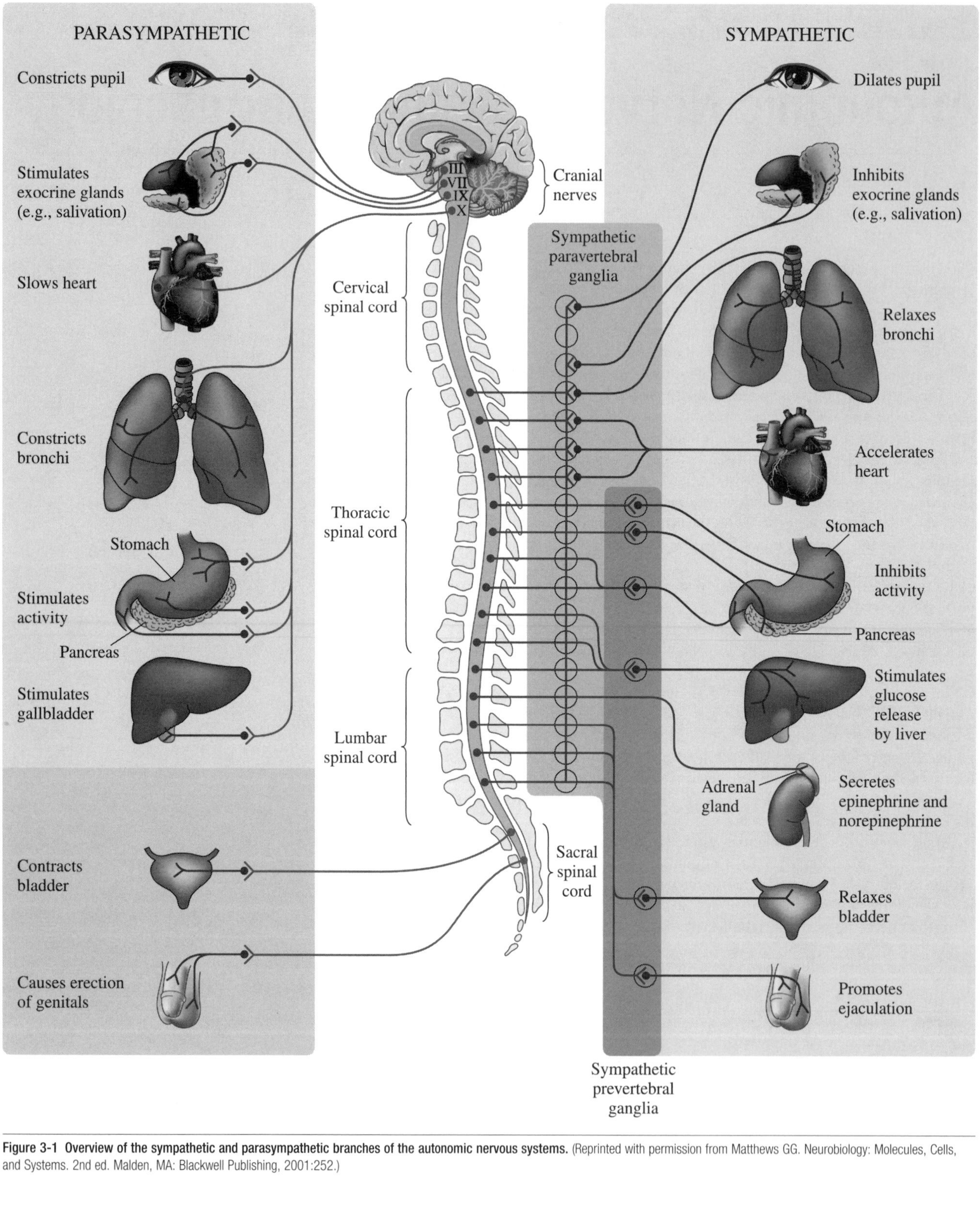

PARASYMPATHETIC

Constricts pupil

Stimulates
exocrine glands
(e.g., salivation)

Slows heart

Constricts
bronchi

Stomach

Stimulates
activity

Pancreas

Stimulates
gallbladder

Contracts
bladder

Causes erection
of genitals

Cranial
nerves

III
VII
IX
X

Cervical
spinal cord

Thoracic
spinal cord

Lumbar
spinal cord

Sacral
spinal
cord

SYMPATHETIC

Dilates pupil

Inhibits
exocrine glands
(e.g., salivation)

Sympathetic
paravertebral
ganglia

Relaxes
bronchi

Accelerates
heart

Stomach

Inhibits
activity

Pancreas

Stimulates
glucose
release
by liver

Adrenal
gland

Secretes
epinephrine and
norepinephrine

Relaxes
bladder

Promotes
ejaculation

Sympathetic
prevertebral
ganglia

Figure 3-1 Overview of the sympathetic and parasympathetic branches of the autonomic nervous systems. (Reprinted with permission from Matthews GG. Neurobiology: Molecules, Cells, and Systems. 2nd ed. Malden, MA: Blackwell Publishing, 2001:252.)

SYMPATHETIC NERVE TERMINAL

PARASYMPATHETIC NERVE TERMINAL

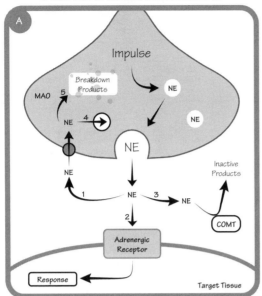
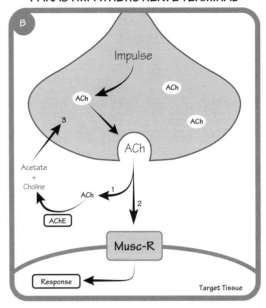

Figure 3-2 Physiology of the sympathetic and parasympathetic nerve terminals. (A) A sympathetic nerve impulse stimulates the release of the neurotransmitter norepinephrine (NE) into the synaptic cleft. Once in the cleft, NE has several possible fates: it can stimulate postsynaptic adrenergic receptors (2); it can be taken back up into the neuron by presynaptic transporters (1); or it can be degraded in the cleft by the enzyme catechol-O-methyltransferase (COMT). NE that is taken back up into the presynaptic neuron can either be reloaded into vesicles (4) and rereleased, or degraded (5) by the enzyme monoamine oxidase (MAO). **(B)** A parasympathetic nerve impulse stimulates the release of the neurotransmitter acetylcholine (ACh) into the synaptic cleft. Once in the cleft, ACh can stimulate postsynaptic muscarinic receptors (1) or be broken down by the enzyme acetylcholinesterase (AChE) to acetate and choline (2). Acetate and choline are taken up by the presynaptic neuron (3) and used to synthesize new ACh.

ENDOGENOUS NEUROTRANSMITTERS

 Acetylcholine

Catecholamines: *Epinephrine, norepinephrine (NE), dopamine*

Acetylcholine

Stimulates both muscarinic and nicotinic cholinergic receptors.

- In the autonomic nervous system, all **preganglionic neurons** release acetylcholine onto **nicotinic receptors** located at the ganglia and on the adrenal medulla.
  - ○ Nicotinic receptors are **ionotropic**, meaning that they produce their effects via alteration of ion channel activity.
- **Postganglionic parasympathetic neurons** also release acetylcholine. **Muscarinic receptors** are located on parasympathetic target organs and are stimulated by acetylcholine released from postganglionic parasympathetic nerve endings.
  - ○ Muscarinic receptors are **metabotropic**, meaning that they are linked to the production of the intracellular second messengers such as 2-diacylglycerol and inositol 1,4,5-trisphosphate.

Catecholamines

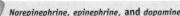 **Norepinephrine, epinephrine, and** *dopamine* **stimulate adrenergic receptors**

The postganglionic sympathetic neurons, with the exception of sweat glands and skeletal muscle blood vessels (see above), release norepinephrine. Several subtypes of postganglionic adrenergic receptors exist, including the **α-adrenergic receptors** and the **β-adrenergic receptors**. Each of these subtypes is further subdivided. The major subtypes of the α-adrenergic receptors are α_1 and α_2, whereas the major subtypes of the β-adrenergic receptors are β_1 and β_2.

- α_1 adrenergic receptors are **metabotropic**, meaning that they are linked to the intracellular production of the second messengers 1,2-diacylglycerol and inositol 1,4,5-trisphosphate.
- α_2, β_1, and β_2 adrenergic receptors are G protein-coupled receptors and are linked to the enzyme **adenylate cyclase**, which, upon activation, produces cyclic AMP (cAMP) from AMP.
- The **adrenal medulla**, which acts as a sympathetic ganglia, releases norepinephrine, epinephrine, and dopamine into the bloodstream.

The distribution and the effect of stimulation of the various autonomic receptors are presented in Table 3-2.

HARDCORE

Several anatomically *sympathetic postganglionic neurons* also release acetylcholine, instead of a typical sympathetic neurotransmitter such as norepinephrine (see below). These include the sympathetic neurons innervating *sweat glands*, as well as sympathetic neurons innervating *skeletal muscle blood vessels*.

TABLE 3-2	Effector Organ Responses to Autonomic Nervous System Stimulation			
EFFECTOR ORGAN	RESPONSE TO PARASYMPATHETIC STIMULATION	RECEPTOR(S) MEDIATING RESPONSE	RESPONSE TO SYMPATHETIC STIMULATION	RECEPTOR(S) MEDIATING RESPONSE
Eyes				
Radial muscle of iris	–	–	Contraction and mydriasis (*large pupils*)	α_1
Sphincter muscle of iris	Contraction and miosis (*small pupils*)	Muscarinic	–	–
Ciliary muscle	Contraction for near vision	Muscarinic	Relaxation for far vision	β_2
GI tract				
Motility	↑	Muscarinic	↓	α_1 and α_2; β_1 and β_2
Secretions	↑	Muscarinic	↓	α_2
Urinary bladder				
Detrusor	Contraction	Muscarinic	Relaxation	β_2
Sphincter	Relaxation	Muscarinic	Contraction	α_1
Skin				
Sweat glands	↑ Secretion	Muscarinic	↑ Secretion	Muscarinic and α_1
Adrenal medulla	–	–	Release of catecholamines	Various adrenergic
Lacrimal glands	Secretion	Muscarinic	Secretion	α
Cardiovascular system				
Heart rate	↓	Muscarinic	↑	β_1 (**1** heart → β_1)
Arterioles	Dilation	Muscarinic	Constriction / dilation	α_1 β_2
Lungs				
Bronchioles	Constrict	Muscarinic	Relaxation	β_2 (**2** lungs → β_2)

DRUGS AFFECTING THE AUTONOMIC NERVOUS SYSTEM

Drugs affecting the autonomic nervous system can be classified according to the type of receptor they target and the effect they have on that receptor (Box 3-1).

Cholinergic Agonists

These drugs produce their effects by activating muscarinic receptors located on effector organs and tissues.

Direct Cholinergic Agonists

> *Bethanechol, carbachol, methacholine, pilocarpine*

Direct cholinergic agonists mimic the actions of acetylcholine by stimulating cholinergic receptors directly.

BETHANECHOL

Indications and Usage—Used to **increase smooth muscle tone**, especially in the GI tract following abdominal surgery or the urinary tract for urinary retention in the absence of obstruction

Mechanism of Action—Stimulates smooth muscle muscarinic receptors, does not stimulate nicotinic receptors

Side Effects—Hypotension, cardiac rate changes, and bronchial spasms

CARBACHOL

Indications and Usage—Used in the eye to produce miosis and to **decrease intraocular pressure in glaucoma**

Mechanism of Action—Stimulates muscarinic receptors on the pupillary sphincter and ciliary muscle of the eye, resulting in opening of Schlemm's canal and drainage of the aqueous humor

Side Effects—None, if used topically

METHACHOLINE

Indications and Usage—Methacholine challenge test for the assessment of airway hyperresponsiveness

HARDCORE

At toxic levels, all cholinergic agonists can cause **generalized cholinergic stimulation**. This effect of excessive cholinergic activation can be remembered by using the mnemonic

SLUDE—Excess **S**alivation, **L**acrimation, **U**rination, **D**efecation, and **E**mesis

HARDCORE

Carbachol stimulates both muscarinic and nicotinic cholinergic receptors, and is resistant to degradation by acetylcholinesterase.

Box 3-1.

Cholinergic Agonists
- Direct agonists: *Bethanechol, carbachol, methacholine, pilocarpine*
- Reversible acetylcholinesterase inhibitors: *Edrophonium, neostigmine, physostigmine, pyridostigmine*
- Irreversible acetylcholinesterase inhibitors: *Isoflurophate, echothiphate, parathion, nerve gases (sarin, VX)*

Cholinergic Antagonists
- Anti-muscarinic agents: *Atropine, ipratropium, scopolamine*
- Ganglionic blockers: *Trimethaphan, hexamethonium*

Adrenergic Agonists
- Direct agonists: *Norepinephrine, epinephrine, isoproterenol, dopamine, dobutamine, albuterol, metaproterenol, terbutaline, phenylephrine, clonidine*
- Indirect-acting agonists: *Amphetamine, cocaine*
- Mixed agonists: *Ephedrine*

Adrenergic Antagonists
- α-blockers: *Prazosin, terazosin, doxazosin, phenoxybenzamine, phentolamine, yohimbine*
- β-blockers: *Pindolol, betaxolol, levobunolol*
- Combined α- and β-blockers: *Labetalol*
- Modulators of neurotransmitter release: *Reserpine, guanethidine*

Additionally, many of the drugs that affect the autonomic nervous system, as well as several other agents, are used to treat disorders of the eye, such as glaucoma:

Ocular Pharmacology (Figure 2-3)
- β-adrenergic receptor blockers: *Timolol, betaxolol, levobunolol*
- Adrenergic agonists: *Epinephrine, dipivefrin, brimonidine*
- Cholinergic agonists: *Pilocarpine, echothiophate, carbachol*
- Carbonic anhydrase inhibitors: *Acetazolamide, dorzolamide*
- Prostaglandin analogs: *Travoprost, latanoprost*
- Hyperosmotic agents: *Glycerin, mannitol*

Mechanism of Action—Stimulation of airway muscarinic smooth muscle receptors, ***resulting in bronchoconstriction***

Side Effects—Airway hyperresponsiveness in asthmatics; excessive cholinergic stimulation, including SLUDE (Salivation, Lacrimation, Urination, Defecation, and Emesis)

PILOCARPINE

Indications and Usage—Open-angle glaucoma, or glaucoma in which the aqueous humor has ***free access to the trabecular meshwork***; radiation-induced xerostomia (dry mouth) in cancer patients

Mechanism of Action—Produces miosis and a reduction of intraocular pressure due to contraction of the pupillary sphincter and the opening of Schlemm's canal respectively; stimulation of salivary secretions

Side Effects—SLUDE

REVERSIBLE ACETYLCHOLINESTERASE INHIBITORS

Edrophonium, neostigmine, physostigmine, pyridostigmine

The enzyme ***acetylcholinesterase*** destroys the neurotransmitter acetylcholine by breaking it down into acetate and choline. This enzyme is located in the synaptic nerve terminal and is responsible for the regulation of levels of acetylcholine. Inhibiting the acetylcholinesterase prevents acetylcholine breakdown, ***indirectly*** increasing the level of cholinergic stimulation. Inhibitors of acetylcholinesterase bind to and inhibit the enzyme for varying durations of time. Some inhibitors bind the enzyme covalently and are essentially ***irreversible***. Irreversible inhibition can only be overcome by the synthesis of a new enzyme. Other inhibitors are ***reversible*** and only bind the enzyme for a period of time, after which the activity of the enzyme is restored.

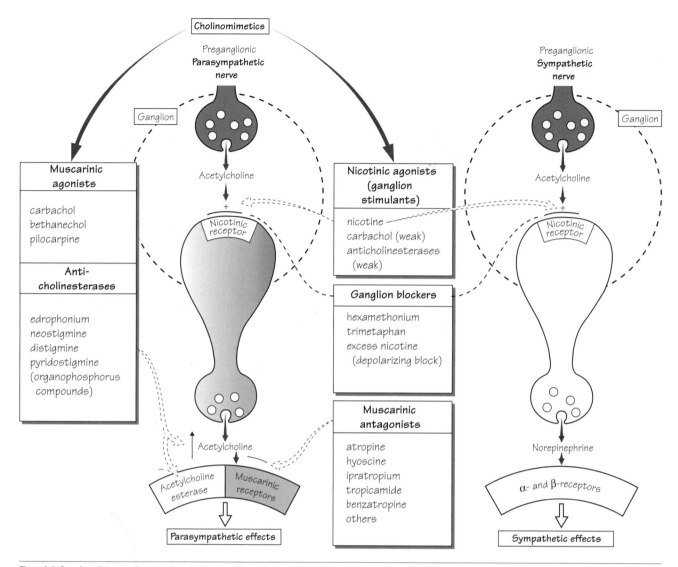

Figure 3-3 Overview of drugs acting at cholinergic synapses. (Reprinted with permission from Neal MJ. Medical Pharmacology at a Glance. 4th ed. Oxford: Blackwell Publishing, 2002:22.)

HARDCORE

Edrophonium has a short duration of action (10 to 20 minutes). If given to a patient with myasthenia gravis, the patient will experience a transient improvement of symptoms due to the *edrophonium*-induced increase in acetylcholine at the skeletal muscle motor endplate. Following diagnosis, patients with myasthenia gravis are treated with neostigmine or pyridostigmine because of their longer duration of action.

HARDCORE

Physostigmine is an uncharged lipophilic molecule and thus can cross the blood-brain barrier, leading to convulsions at high doses. For this reason, it is not used for treatment of myasthenia gravis.

EDROPHONIUM

Indications and Usage—***Diagnosis of myasthenia gravis***; antidote for nondepolarizing muscle relaxants (e.g., *tubocurarine*)

Mechanism of Action—Reversible inhibition of acetylcholinesterase

Side Effects—Signs of generalized cholinergic stimulation, including SLUDE and bradycardia

PHYSOSTIGMINE

Indications and Usage—Overdose of atropine or tricyclic antidepressants (potent anticholinergic side effects; see Chapter 2), intestinal immotility

Mechanism of Action—***Reversible inhibition of acetylcholinesterase***

Side Effects—SLUDE; seizures if given rapidly intravenously; bradycardia; paralysis at high doses

NEOSTIGMINE AND PYRIDOSTIGMINE

Indications and Usage—Postoperative gastric distention, urinary retention, ***myasthenia gravis***; antidote for nondepolarizing muscle relaxants (e.g., *tubocurarine*)

Mechanism of Action—Reversible inhibition of acetylcholinesterase

Side Effects—Signs of generalized cholinergic stimulation, including SLUDE, bronchospasm, skeletal muscle paralysis, respiratory depression, and AV block; skin rash and thrombophlebitis can occur after intravenous administration of *pyridostigmine*

Irreversible Acetylcholinesterase Inhibitors

These drugs irreversibly inhibit acetylcholinesterase.

ISOFLUROPHATE (also known as diisopropylfluorophosphate [DFP])

Indications and Usage—Chronic treatment of open-angle glaucoma

Mechanism of Action—***Irreversible inhibition of acetylcholinesterase***; causes intense miosis due to stimulation of the pupillary sphincter of the eye, and thereby ***increases aqueous humor outflow***

Side Effects—SLUDE, bradycardia, visual disturbances, muscle weakness and twitching, respiratory distress, seizures, coma

NERVE GASES

The nerve gases, including *sarin* and *VX*, are ***irreversible inhibitors of acetylcholinesterase***. *VX* is one of the most toxic substances known. These agents have no clinical use, and are discussed further in Chapter 12.

Cholinergic Antagonists

Antimuscarinic agents: *Atropine, ipratropium, scopolamine*

Ganglionic blockers: *Trimethaphan, hexamethonium*

Cholinergic antagonists bind directly to cholinergic receptors, but are not able to stimulate the receptors. Drugs within this class are capable of blocking either ganglionic impulses or parasympathetic impulses at the effector organ or tissue.

Antimuscarinic Agents

Atropine, ipratropium, scopolamine

These agents block muscarinic receptors located at effector organs and tissues.

ATROPINE

Indications and Usage—Excessive muscarinic stimulation, such as following intoxication with an acetylcholinesterase inhibitor, bradycardia, block of secretions prior to surgery

Mechanism of Action—Competitive blockade of muscarinic receptors

Side Effects—Tachycardia; generalized cholinergic blockade

IPRATROPIUM

Indications and Usage—Asthma and chronic obstructive pulmonary disease (inhaled form; see Chapter 6 for more detail)

Mechanism of Action—Blockade of muscarinic receptors, resulting in a ***reduction in bronchiolar secretions and bronchiolar constriction***

Side Effects—Rare if inhaled, tachycardia

SCOPOLAMINE

Indications and Usage—Motion sickness; short-term memory blockade

Mechanism of Action—Blockade of muscarinic receptors

Side Effects—Generalized cholinergic blockade

Ganglionic Blockers

Nicotine, trimethaphan, hexamethonium

These agents block nicotinic receptors at autonomic ganglia. Because both sympathetic and parasympathetic ganglionic impulses are mediated by nicotinic receptors, these agents block activity in both branches of the autonomic nervous system (Table 3-3 and Figure 3-4).

NICOTINE

Indications and Usage—No clinical uses, but is a dangerous component of cigarette smoke

Mechanism of Action—Initial stimulation of nicotinic receptors, followed by desensitization

Side Effects—Drop in blood pressure, irritability, tremors, withdrawal syndromes, increased drug metabolism

TRIMETHAPHAN AND HEXAMETHONIUM

Indications and Usage—Situations requiring a rapid decrease in blood pressure, such as pulmonary edema or dissecting aortic aneurysm

Mechanism of Action—Blockade of nicotinic receptors at autonomic ganglia, resulting in a loss of sympathetic tone to blood vessels and a decrease in blood pressure

Side Effects—Hypotension

HARDCORE

Neostigmine is the drug of choice for myasthenia gravis because it has a longer half-life than *physostigmine* (decreased daily dosing) and does not cross the blood-brain barrier (does not have CNS side effects).

HARDCORE

Isoflurophate is extremely potent as a toxin. It is the prototype of many insecticides and the nerve gases.

HARDCORE

Pralidoxime (also known as 2-PAM) is a synthetic compound that is able to reactivate acetylcholinesterase that has been inhibited by *isoflurophate* or its derivatives. However, *pralidoxime* must be given before "*aging*" of the isoflurophate-acetylcholinesterase complex occurs. "*Aging*" refers to the loss of an alkyl group, which makes the bond between *isoflurophate* and the enzyme too strong to break.

HARDCORE

Blockade of cardiac muscarinic receptors with atropine allows unopposed sympathetic stimulation of the heart and results in an increase in heart rate. Therefore, atropine can be used to increase heart rate in patients with bradycardia.

HARDCORE

At toxic doses, atropine and other muscarinic antagonists can cause ***generalized cholinergic blockage***. These anticholinergic side effects include the following:

- **Blind as a bat**—Blocks the ability of the pupil to constrict, resulting in mydriasis and the inability to focus for near vision (cycloplegia)
- **Red as a beet**—Causes dilation of the cutaneous vasculature
- **Mad as a hatter**—Acts on the CNS causing restlessness, confusion, and delirium
- **Dry as a bone**—Blocks salivary, lacrimal, and sweat glands
- **Hot as hell**—Elevates body temperature

HARDCORE

Table 3-3 indicates the dominant branch of the autonomic nervous system in each organ system at rest and the effect that ganglionic blockade would have on each system.

TABLE 3-3	Effect of Ganglionic Blockade	
TISSUE OR ORGAN SYSTEM	DOMINANT BRANCH OF THE ANS	EFFECT OF GANGLIONIC BLOCKADE
Heart	Parasympathetic	Tachycardia
Arteries / veins	Sympathetic	Vasodilation
Eyes	Parasympathetic	Mydriasis
GI tract	Parasympathetic	Immotility / constipation
Genitourinary	Parasympathetic	Urinary retention

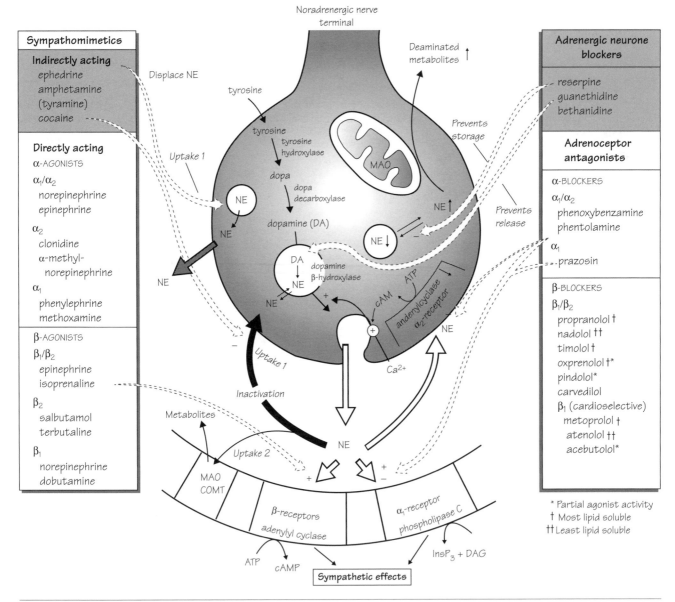

Figure 3-4 Overview of drugs that act on the sympathetic nervous system. (Reprinted with permission from Neal MJ. Medical Pharmacology at a Glance. 4th ed. Oxford: Blackwell Publishing, 2002:24.)

Adrenergic Agonists (also known as *Sympathomimetics*)

Adrenergic receptors are endogenously activated by the catecholamines, including *norepinephrine* and *epinephrine*. Drugs within this class are able to stimulate adrenergic receptors, either directly or indirectly.

Direct Adrenergic Agonists (Nonselective and selective α and β)
These agents activate adrenergic receptors directly.

  Nonselective α- and β-adrenergic receptor agonists (*norepinephrine, epinephrine*)

NOREPINEPHRINE

Receptors Stimulated—α_1, α_2, β_1 ($\alpha > \beta$)

Indications and Usage—Shock (becoming first-line therapy because of best efficacy)

Mechanism of Action—At therapeutic doses, *norepinephrine* primarily **stimulates α-adrenergic receptors** (increasing both systolic and diastolic blood pressure while narrowing pulse pressure). With increasing concentrations, *norepinephrine* will stimulate β_1 receptors, increasing heart rate and contractility.

Side Effects—Tissue (e.g., kidney and others) hypoperfusion and necrosis secondary to vasoconstriction, elevated blood pressure, tachycardia, hemorrhage, arrhythmias

EPINEPHRINE

Receptors Stimulated—α_1, α_2, β_1, β_2

Indications and Usage

- Emergent treatment of bronchoconstriction due to asthma or anaphylactic shock
- Hypotension due to sepsis, hemorrhage, or neurogenic shock
- Glaucoma
- Adjunct for local anesthesia

Mechanism of Action—*Epinephrine* can **stimulate both α and β receptors, but at low doses β effects predominate** (*vasodilation, heart rate,* and *myocardial contractility*), resulting in an increased systolic pressure, decreased diastolic pressure, and widened pulse pressure. As *epinephrine* concentrations increase, α receptors are stimulated, resulting in *vasoconstriction*.

Side Effects—Anxiety, headache, tremor, hemorrhage, arrhythmias

 Selective α-adrenergic receptor agonists (*phenylephrine, clonidine*)

PHENYLEPHRINE

Receptors Stimulated—Selective for α-adrenergic receptors ($\alpha_1 > \alpha_2$)

Indications and Usage—Nasal congestion

Mechanism of Action—**Stimulates α_1 receptors**, resulting in vasoconstriction in the nasal mucous membranes and reduced secretions

Side Effects—Hypertensive headache and cardiac irregularities

CLONIDINE

Receptors Stimulated—Selective for α_2 receptors

Indications and Usage—Hypertension, neurodepressant withdrawal (opiates and benzodiazepines)

Mechanism of Action—Acts on **α_2-adrenergic receptors in the CNS** to increase the α_2–mediated negative feedback on norepinephrine release in the presynaptic nerve terminal, resulting in a decrease in sympathetic vascular tone

Side Effects—Sexual dysfunction, orthostatic hypotension, nausea, headache

 Selective β-adrenergic receptor agonists (*isoproterenol, albuterol, metaproterenol, terbutaline*)

ISOPROTERENOL

Receptors Stimulated—β-adrenergic receptors

Indications and Usage—Shock (rarely used), bradycardia

Mechanism of Action—**Equal activation of all β-adrenergic receptor isotypes.** Stimulation of β_2 adrenergic receptor results in vasodilation of skeletal muscle arterioles (*hypotension*); stimulation of β_1 adrenergic receptors results in an increase in heart rate and contractility.

Side Effects—Tremor, palpitations, hemorrhage, arrhythmias

ALBUTEROL, METAPROTERENOL, TERBUTALINE

See Chapter 6 for a more extensive discussion.

Receptors Stimulated—Selective for β_2-adrenergic receptors

Indications and Usage—Asthma, chronic obstructive pulmonary disease (COPD), bronchospasm

Mechanism of Action—**Selective stimulation of β_2-adrenergic receptors**

Side Effects—Rare if the inhaled formulation is used; if administered systemically, tachycardia and hypotension can occur

Dopamine Receptor Agonists

 Dopamine, dobutamine

HARDCORE

Stimulation of dopamine D-1 receptors in peripheral mesenteric and renal vascular beds results in vasodilation.

HARDCORE

Stimulation of dopamine D-2 receptors on presynaptic adrenergic neurons decreases norepinephrine release.

HARDCORE

Dobutamine is used for cardiac stress testing, because the drug increases cardiac output without greatly elevating oxygen demands of the myocardium, an important consideration in patients with limited myocardial oxygen capacity.

HARDCORE

Termination of the actions of norepinephrine is primarily due to reuptake into the presynaptic neuron. Within the presynaptic neuron, norepinephrine can be reloaded in vesicles or broken down by the enzyme monoamine oxidase (MAO).

HARDCORE

Never use a β-blocker (e.g., *propranolol*) for *cocaine*-induced hypertension because of the resulting unopposed alpha-adrenergic receptor stimulation and subsequent coronary vasoconstriction that occur.

DOPAMINE

Receptors Stimulated—β-adrenergic, α-adrenergic, dopamine (DA) (DA > β > α)

Indications and Usage—**Shock**; acute renal failure

Mechanism of Action—Stimulates both adrenergic and dopaminergic receptors:

- Lower doses stimulate mainly *dopaminergic receptors* and produce renal and mesenteric vasodilation.
- Medium doses stimulate both *dopaminergic and β_1 adrenergic receptors* and produce cardiac stimulation and renal vasodilation.
- Larger doses stimulate *α-adrenergic receptors*.

Side Effects—Nausea, hypertension, arrhythmias

DOBUTAMINE

Receptors Stimulated—β-adrenergic receptors ($\beta_1 \gg \beta_2$)

Indications and Usage—Cardiac stress tests, decompensated congestive heart failure (CHF)

Mechanism of Action—*Selectively stimulates β_1-adrenergic receptors*, resulting in increased heart rate and contractility

Side Effects—Increases AV nodal conduction (use with caution in patients with atrial fibrillation), tachycardia, tremor

Indirect Adrenergic Agonists

 Amphetamine, cocaine

AMPHETAMINE

Receptors Stimulated—α- and β-adrenergic receptors, both peripherally and centrally

Indications and Usage—Narcolepsy, **attention deficit and hyperactivity disorder (ADHD)**, appetite suppression in obese patients

Mechanism of Action—*Releases norepinephrine from presynaptic neurons*, resulting in increased levels of catecholamines in the synaptic space

Side Effects—Insomnia, irritability, arrhythmias, hypertension

COCAINE

Receptors Stimulated—α- and β-adrenergic receptors, both peripheral and central

Indications and Usage—Local anesthesia for dental and ear, nose, and throat (ENT) surgical procedures

Mechanism of Action—*Blocks the reuptake of catecholamines into the presynaptic neuron*, resulting in increased levels of catecholamines in the synaptic space

Side Effects—Hypertension, tachycardia, paranoia, depression, seizure, arrhythmias, addiction (*cocaine is one of the most addictive substances known*)

Mixed Adrenergic Agonists

These agents stimulate adrenergic receptors both directly and indirectly.

EPHEDRINE

Receptors Stimulated—β_2 directly; nonselective indirect stimulation of peripheral α- and β-receptors

Indications and Usage—Nasal decongestant

Mechanism of Action—Induces the release of NE from presynaptic neurons and activates β_2 receptors directly

Side Effects—Arrhythmias, hyperactivity, insomnia, tremors

Adrenergic Antagonists

Prazosin, terazosin, doxazosin, phenoxybenzamine, phentolamine, yohimbine

Adrenergic antagonists have affinity for adrenergic receptors, but do not possess intrinsic activity at those receptors, effectively blocking endogenous activity at the receptor. There are several classes of adrenergic antagonists. Each class is outlined below, along with the commonly used drugs from each class. Since these drugs are mainly used to treat cardiovascular diseases, details about each drug are presented in Chapter 4.

α-Adrenergic Receptor Blockers

α-adrenergic receptors are most commonly used to lower blood pressure, since α_1 adrenergic receptors play a significant role in modulating vascular tone.

β-Adrenergic Receptor Blockers

 Propranolol, timolol, nadolol, metoprolol, atenolol, esmolol, acebutolol, pindolol

Drugs in this class block β-adrenergic receptor activation. These drugs are commonly used to lower blood pressure, but can also be employed to control heart rate, treat angina, and eliminate cardiac arrhythmias.

Combined α- and β-Adrenergic Receptor Blockers

 Labetalol

This class of drugs is used for acute hypertension and tachycardia in hospital settings.

Modulators of Neurotransmitter Release

 Reserpine, guanethidine

These drugs act within the presynaptic neuron to limit the release of neurotransmitters from storage vesicles. These agents are rarely used today (except in Step 1 questions) due to their significant side effects, and are covered in Chapter 4, Cardiovascular Pharmacology.

Ocular Pharmacology

 β-adrenergic receptor blockers: *Timolol, betaxolol, levobunolol*

Adrenergic agonists: *Epinephrine, dipivefrin, brimonidine*

Cholinergic agonists: *Pilocarpine, echothiophate, carbachol*

Carbonic anhydrase inhibitors: *Acetazolamide, dorzolamide*

Prostaglandin analogs: *Travoprost, latanoprost*

Hyperosmotic agents: *Glycerin, mannitol*

Ocular pharmacologic agents focus primarily on the treatment of glaucoma. Glaucoma is a pathologic increase in intraocular pressure that, if untreated, can result in gradual optic nerve damage and subsequent loss of vision. There are two primary types of glaucoma: open-angle glaucoma and closed-angle glaucoma ("angle" refers to the filtration angle formed between the iris and cornea). Open-angle glaucoma is a chronic disease caused by diminished drainage of the aqueous humor through the canal of Schlemm. Closed-angle glaucoma is an emergent situation that results from a ballooning peripheral iris that reduces the flow of aqueous humor between the cornea and iris. Treatment of glaucoma is directed at lowering intraocular pressure by either:

HARDCORE

Aqueous humor formation can also be reduced by activating α_1 receptors, which constrict ciliary vessels and limit ciliary blood flow.

- *Decreasing aqueous humor inflow (production)*: Aqueous humor production is *stimulated by β_1 receptors and inhibited by α_2 receptors*, both located on the ocular ciliary body. Production of aqueous humor depends on the active transport of bicarbonate and sodium ions, so reducing the activity of carbonic anhydrase also diminishes aqueous humor production.

- *Increasing aqueous humor outflow*: Cholinergic agonists activate muscarinic receptors, constricting ciliary muscles and resulting in a more spherical lens shape. This change in lens shape allows for an increased aqueous humor outflow.

Figure 3-5 depicts physiological regulation of the eye.

Some of the agents listed below have been covered in previous sections, but are repeated here to emphasize their ocular effects. Other agents listed above affect systems that are not traditionally considered to be part of the autonomic nervous system. However, in the eye, many of these systems play a role in the unconscious control of intraocular pressure, and, therefore, we include them with drugs acting on the ANS.

β-Adrenergic Receptor Blockers: β_1

 Timolol, betaxolol, levobunolol

Indications and Usage—Open-angle glaucoma

Mechanism of Action—β-adrenergic receptor blockade results in decreased inflow of aqueous humor.

Side Effects—Dry eyes, blurred vision, blepharitis

Adrenergic Agonists

EPINEPHRINE: α_1

Indications and Usage—Open-angle glaucoma

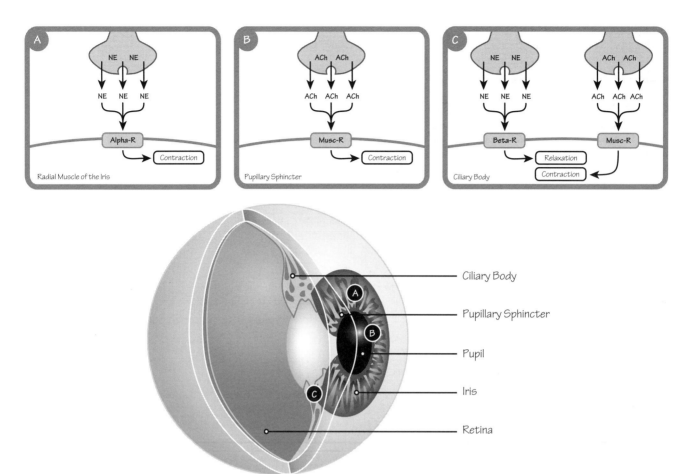

Figure 3-5 Physiological regulation of the eye. (A) Stimulation of α-adrenergic receptors located on the radial muscle of the iris by norepinephrine (NE) released from adrenergic neurons results in constriction of the muscle and mydriasis. **(B)** Stimulation of muscarinic receptors (R-Mus) located on the pupillary sphincter by acetylcholine (ACh) released from parasympathetic neurons results in pupil constriction (miosis). **(C)** Stimulation of β-adrenergic receptors located on the ciliary muscle by NE released from sympathetic neurons results in relaxation of the muscle and formation of aqueous humor. Stimulation of muscarinic receptors located on the ciliary muscle results in contraction of the muscle and outflow of aqueous humor through the canal of Schlemm.

Mechanism of Action—Reduces the production of aqueous humor by **constricting blood vessels in the ciliary body**

Side Effects—Mydriasis, burning in the eyes, conjunctival hyperemia

Brimonidine: α₂

Indications and Usage—Open-angle glaucoma

Mechanism of Action—α_2-adrenergic receptor stimulation results in decreased inflow of aqueous humor

Side Effects—Allergic reactions, including edema, hyperemia, and itching

Cholinergic Agonists

 Pilocarpine, echothiophate, carbachol

Indications and Usage—Closed-angle glaucoma

Mechanism of Action—Increases aqueous outflow secondary to muscarinic receptor stimulation

Side Effects—Miosis, cataracts, periorbital pain

Carbonic Anhydrase Inhibitors

 Acetazolamide, dichlorphenamide, dorzolamide

Indications and Usage—Closed-angle and open-angle glaucoma; metabolic alkalosis

Mechanism of Action—**Reversibly inhibits the enzyme carbonic anhydrase**. In the eye, this results in a reduction in the amount of bicarbonate secreted into the aqueous humor and a decrease in intraocular pressure. In the kidneys, inhibition of carbonic anhydrase results in a reduction in the amount of bicarbonate reabsorbed in the proximal tubule.

Side Effects—Myopia, flushing, tinnitus

HARDCORE

Acetazolamide is contraindicated in patients with sulfa allergies.

Prostaglandin Analogs

 Travoprost, latanoprost

Indications and Usage—Open-angle glaucoma

Mechanism of Action—Selective prostanoid receptor agonist that increases fluid outflow thereby lowering intraocular pressure

Side Effects—Conjunctival hyperemia, iris pigmentation, blurry vision

Hyperosmotic Agents

 Glycerin, mannitol

Indications and Usage—Closed-angle glaucoma

Mechanism of Action—Creates an **osmotic gradient** between the plasma and aqueous humor, resulting in movement of fluid out of the eye and a decrease in intraocular pressure

Side Effects—Headache, diuresis, dehydration

HARDCORE

For closed-angle glaucoma, *glycerin* is the oral drug of choice, and *mannitol* is the intravenous drug of choice.

HARDCORE REVIEW – ANS PHARMACOLOGY

HARDCORE Side Effects

Remember these important side effects:

Cholinergic Agonists

- **SLUDE**—Excess Salivation, Lacrimation, Urination, Defecation, and Emesis

Anticholinergic Agents

- **Blind as a bat**—Blocks the ability of the pupil to constrict, resulting in mydriasis and the inability to focus for near vision (cycloplegia)
- **Red as a beet**—Causes dilation of the cutaneous vasculature
- **Mad as a hatter**—Acts on the CNS, causing restlessness, confusion, and delirium
- **Dry as a bone**—Blocks salivary, lacrimal, and sweat glands
- **Hot as hell (Hardcore)**—Elevates body temperature

TABLE 3-4 Cholinergic Agonists

DRUG CLASS	DRUGS	MECHANISM OF ACTION	MAJOR SIDE EFFECTS
Direct acting	Bethanechol	Activates muscarinic receptors in the bladder	SLUDE
	Carbachol	Activates muscarinic receptors on ciliary bodies of the eye	If topical, rare
	Pilocarpine	Muscarinic activation on ciliary bodies	CNS manifestations, SLUDE
Indirect and reversible	Edrophonium	Acetylcholinesterase enzyme inhibitor	SLUDE
	Neostigmine	Acetylcholinesterase enzyme inhibitor	SLUDE
	Physostigmine	Acetylcholinesterase enzyme inhibitor	SLUDE
	Pyridostigmine	Acetylcholinesterase enzyme inhibitor	SLUDE
Indirect and irreversible	Echothiophate	Acetylcholinesterase enzyme inhibitor	SLUDE, bradycardia, death
	Pralidoxime	Reactivates inhibited acetylcholinesterase	

TABLE 3-5 Cholinergic Antagonists

DRUG CLASS	DRUGS	MECHANISM OF ACTION	MAJOR SIDE EFFECTS
Antimuscarinic	Atropine	Blocks muscarinic receptors	Anticholinergic
	Ipratropium	Blocks muscarinic-mediated bronchiole constriction/secretions	Rare if inhaled
	Scopolamine	Blocks muscarinic receptors	Anticholinergic
Ganglionic blockers	Nicotine	Ganglionic nicotinic receptor blocker	Hypotension, irritability, tremors, increased drug metabolism
	Trimethaphan	Ganglionic nicotinic receptor blocker	Hypotension

TABLE 3-6 Adrenergic Agonists

Drug Class	Drugs	Mechanism of Action	Major Side Effects
Direct-acting	Norepinephrine	α_1, α_2, β_1 ($\alpha > \beta$)	Hypertension, tachycardia, hemorrhage, arrhythmias
	Epinephrine	α_1, α_2, β_1, β_2	Anxiety, hypertension, hemorrhage, arrhythmias
	Phenylephrine	α receptors ($\alpha_1 > \alpha_2$)	Hypertensive headache
	Clonidine	Central (CNS) α_2 receptors	Headache, nausea
	Albuterol	β_2 selective	Rare if inhaled
	Metaproterenol	β_2 selective	Rare if inhaled
	Terbutaline	β_2 selective	Rare if inhaled
	Dopamine	β, α- and dopamine (D-1 = D-2 > β > α)	Hypertension, arrhythmias
	Dobutamine	β-receptors ($\beta_1 > \beta_2$)	Tachycardia (increases AVN conduction)
Indirect-acting	Amphetamine	α, β, CNS: Releases presynaptic NE and inhibits MAO	Insomnia, irritability, arrhythmias, hypertension
	Cocaine	α, β, CNS: Reuptake inhibitor	Hypertension, tachycardia, paranoia, depression, seizure, arrhythmias, death
Mixed	Ephedrine	α, β, CNS: Induces the release of NE from presynaptic neurons and activates adrenergic receptors directly	Arrhythmias, hyperactivity, insomnia, tremors

TABLE 3-7 Adrenergic Antagonists

Drug Class	Drugs	Mechanism of Action	Major Side Effects
α-Blockers	Prazosin, terazosin, doxazosin	α_1 selective	Fatigue, nasal congestion, orthostatic hypotension
	Phenoxybenzamine	Irreversible nonselective α-blocker—α_1 and α_2	Postural hypotension, tachycardia, anginal pain
	Phentolamine	Reversible nonselective α-blocker—α_1 and α_2	Arrhythmias, tachycardia, anginal pain
	Yohimbine	α_2–Blocker	Tachycardia, tremor
β-Blockers	Propranolol	Nonselective β-blocker—β_1 and β_2	Bronchoconstriction, bradycardia, impotence
	Timolol, nadolol	Nonselective β-blocker—β_1 and β_2	Bronchoconstriction, bradycardia, impotence
	Metoprolol, atenolol, esmolol	Selective β_1 blocker	Arrhythmias, sexual dysfunction, depression
	Acebutolol, pindolol	Nonselective partial β-agonists/antagonists	Bronchoconstriction, bradycardia, impotence
Combined α- and β-blockers	Labetalol	Reversibly blocks β receptors (β_1 and 2) while concurrently blocking α_1 receptors	Orthostatic hypotension, bronchoconstriction, bradycardia, impotence
Neurotransmitter release	Reserpine	Blocks the transport of amines from neuronal cytoplasm into storage vesicles	Hypotension, bradycardia, syncope
	Guanethidine	Blocks the storage vesicle release of catecholamines from presynaptic nerve terminals	Hypotension, impotence, syncope

TABLE 3-8 Ocular/Glaucoma Pharmacology

Drug Class	Drugs	Mechanism of Action	Major Side Effects
β-Blockers	Timolol, betolol, levobunolol	Decreases aqueous inflow	Dry eyes and blurred vision
α_2 Agonists	Brimonidine	Decreases aqueous inflow	Allergic reactions
Carbonic anhydrase inhibitors	Acetazolamide, dorzolamide	Decreases aqueous inflow	Conjunctivitis, photophobia
Sympathomimetics	Epinephrine, dipivefrin	Increases aqueous outflow	Conjunctival hyperemia
Parasympathomimetics	Pilocarpine, echothiophate, carbachol	Increases aqueous outflow	Periorbital pain
Prostaglandin analogs	Travoprost, latanoprost	Increases aqueous outflow	Conjunctival hyperemia, iris pigmentation
Hyperosmotic agents	Glycerin, mannitol	Osmotic gradient reduces intraocular fluid	Dehydration

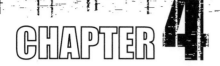

CHAPTER 4

Cardiovascular and Renal Pharmacology

Cardiovascular pharmacology is extensively tested on the USMLE Step 1, due in large part to the tremendous incidence of cardiovascular disease commonly seen in the clinical setting. It is very important that you master the concepts presented in this chapter. Understanding the pathologic basis of the commonly seen cardiovascular diseases is essential to answering board questions regarding cardiovascular pharmacology.

DISEASES OF THE CARDIOVASCULAR SYSTEM (THE BASICS)

Hypertension

Hypertension is defined as a sustained systolic pressure > 140 mm Hg or a diastolic pressure > 90 mm Hg. A systolic blood pressure > 130 mm Hg and/or a diastolic pressure > 85 mm Hg is considered **prehypertension or high-normal blood pressure**. Of patients with hypertension, 95% have **essential, or primary, hypertension**, which refers to high blood pressure with no identifiable cause. The remaining 5% of patients can be classified as having **secondary hypertension**, which refers to high blood pressure caused by a clinically identifiable reason, such as renal disease or pheochromocytoma.

Although individuals with hypertension often do not have any symptoms, chronic high blood pressure can progress to more serious cardiovascular conditions, including heart failure, myocardial infarction (MI), kidney damage, and vascular abnormalities. For patients with secondary hypertension, the treatment is aimed at alleviating the underlying condition. The primary goal of treatment for essential hypertension is to restore blood pressure to a normal level by *reducing peripheral vascular resistance, cardiac output, or fluid retention*. The major drug classes used to treat hypertension include:

- Diuretics
- Sympatholytics
- Angiotensin antagonists
- Calcium channel blockers
- Vasodilating agents

Angina Pectoris

This term literally means "chest pain," and typically occurs during physical activity or emotional stress. This pain is generally substernal, and may radiate from the thorax to the jaw or either shoulder. Angina pectoris occurs during periods of *transient ischemia* in myocardial tissue when coronary vessels are unable to supply enough oxygenated blood to meet the demands of the heart. There are two types of angina pectoris:

- *Exertional angina pectoris (typical or "stable")*: Occurs during strenuous activity when diseased and stenosed coronary arteries are unable to supply enough blood to meet the oxygen demand of the myocardium. Exertional angina pectoris typically subsides once the strenuous activity ceases, and myocardial oxygen demand is reduced.

- *Resting angina pectoris (atypical)*: Chest pain that occurs at rest. There are two types of resting angina pectoris:

  ○ <u>Unstable angina</u>—Similar to stable angina, in that it is due to coronary luminal narrowing; however, the chest pain of unstable angina can occur spontaneously either at rest or during activity. Typically this is a very serious prognostic indicator suggestive of an impending myocardial infarction.

  ○ <u>Prinzmetal's, or variant, angina</u>—Classically occurs at night while the patient is sleeping. This variant is due to spontaneous vasospasm in the coronary arterial system.

Treatment for angina pectoris is directed at improving coronary blood supply to the heart while limiting myocardial demand. Classes of drugs used include:

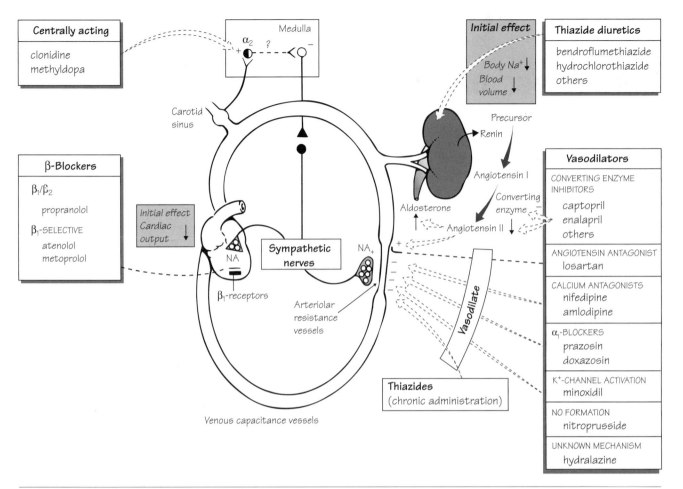

Figure 4-1 Drugs used to treat hypertension. (Reprinted with permission from Neal MJ. Medical Pharmacology at a Glance. 4th ed. Oxford: Blackwell Publishing, 2002:36.)

- Sympatholytics
- Vasodilators
- Diuretics
- Calcium channel blockers
- Anticoagulants

Heart Failure

The term "heart failure" refers to a condition in which the heart is unable to pump enough blood to meet the metabolic demands of the body. Most commonly, the left ventricle fails to generate enough contractile force to effectively pump blood into the aorta against the peripheral vascular pressure. Fluid then backs up from the left ventricle into the pulmonary system, resulting in an increased pulmonary venous volume and edema. When this occurs, the condition is referred to as **congestive heart failure (CHF)**. In right ventricular failure, fluid may back up from the right heart into the systemic venous system, resulting in an increased venous volume. This increase in systemic venous volume can result in lower limb edema, liver congestion, and increased portal pressures.

Heart failure can be further classified as either systolic or diastolic failure, depending on which component of the cardiac cycle is dysfunctional. **Systolic dysfunction** occurs when the heart is unable to generate enough contractile force during systole to pump enough blood to meet the metabolic needs of the body. Systolic dysfunction is typically secondary to myocardial injury caused by myocardial infarction or insufficient coronary blood flow. **Diastolic dysfunction** occurs when the ventricle is unable to relax sufficiently to allow the necessary amount of blood to enter. This commonly occurs in cases of ventricular hypertrophy following chronic hypertension.

The body has several mechanisms by which it attempts to compensate for the diminished cardiac output that occurs in heart failure (Figure 4-3). In compensated heart failure, these mechanisms are able to restore cardiac output to normal. In uncompensated heart failure, the compensatory mechanisms are unable to restore cardiac output to normal.

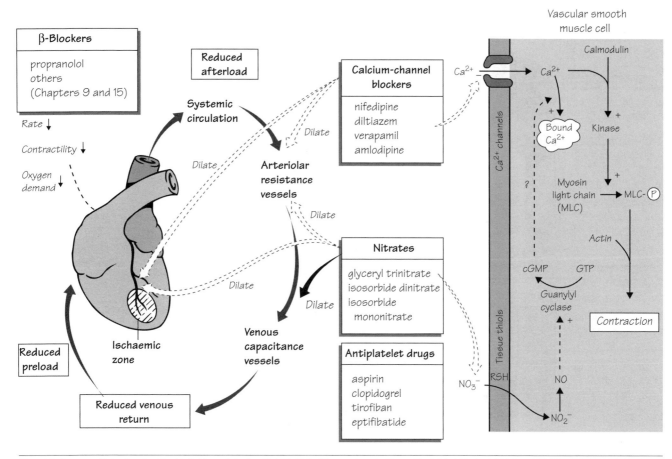

Figure 4-2 Drugs used to treat angina. (Reprinted with permission from Neal MJ. Medical Pharmacology at a Glance. 4th ed. Oxford: Blackwell Publishing, 2002:38.)

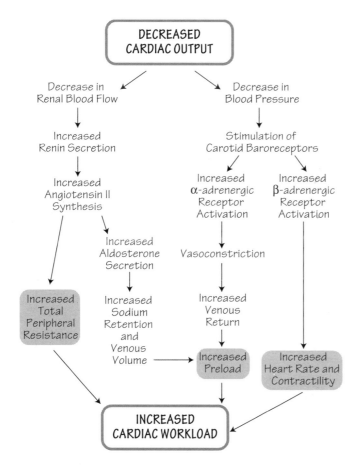

Figure 4-3 Compensatory mechanisms in heart failure. A decrease in cardiac output results in a drop in blood pressure that is sensed by the carotid baroreceptors, leading to activation of the sympathetic nervous system. Sympathetic activation results in both an increase in heart rate through β_1-receptor stimulation in the heart and total peripheral resistance through α_1-receptor stimulation in blood vessels. This increase in total peripheral resistance results in increased venous return and an increase in the preload on the heart. Thus, the net result of sympathetic stimulation is to increase the workload on the heart. Decreased cardiac output also results in a decrease in renal blood flow, resulting in renin release. Increased renin levels result in increased angiotensin II and aldosterone synthesis, resulting in an increase in total peripheral resistance and Na^+ retention, respectively. Both of these effects increase venous volume, resulting in an increased preload on the heart. Over time, due to the increased workload on the heart, the body's compensatory mechanisms actually potentiate the cardiologic failure they are trying to correct.

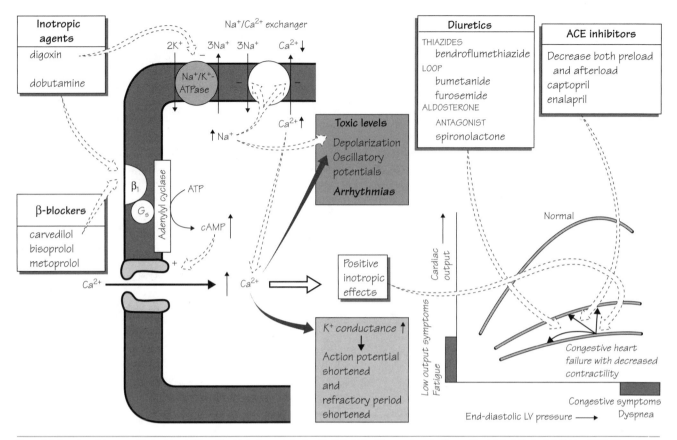

Figure 4-4 **Overview of drugs used to treat heart failure.** (Reprinted with permission from Neal MJ. Medical Pharmacology at a Glance. 4th ed. Oxford: Blackwell Publishing, 2002:42.)

Goals of treatment for heart failure are aimed at increasing cardiac output and reducing the workload of the heart. Therefore, agents that reduce the workload on the heart and decrease total peripheral resistance are often employed:

- Vasodilators
- Diuretics
- Inotropic agents
- β-blockers (in patients with stable CHF)

Lipid Disorders

Hyperlipidemia is a multifactorial disease characterized by elevated blood cholesterol (i.e., the low-density lipoprotein [LDL] component) and/or triglycerides (TGs). Clinically, this disorder is attributed as a major risk factor in the development of coronary artery disease (CAD). To better understand lipid disorders and the drugs used to treat them, a good grasp of the lipoprotein components of the blood (Table 4-1) and their physiologic role in the body is necessary:

- **Chylomicrons (CMs):** Dietary lipids are absorbed and assembled within intestinal mucosal cells into CMs. CMs are rich in TGs and contain the cellular marker apoC-II, which interacts with the adipose cell enzyme *lipoprotein lipase*. Lipoprotein lipase degrades TGs and

TABLE 4-1	Lipoprotein Components of the Blood
LIPOPROTEIN	**MAIN FUNCTION**
CMs	Deliver fatty acids as part of a triglyceride from diet to the periphery
CM remnants	Deliver cholesterol to liver
VLDL	Deliver triglycerides from liver to the periphery
LDL	From VLDL, delivers cholesterol from the liver to the periphery
HDL	Scavenges cholesterol from extra-hepatic tissue and delivers it back to the liver

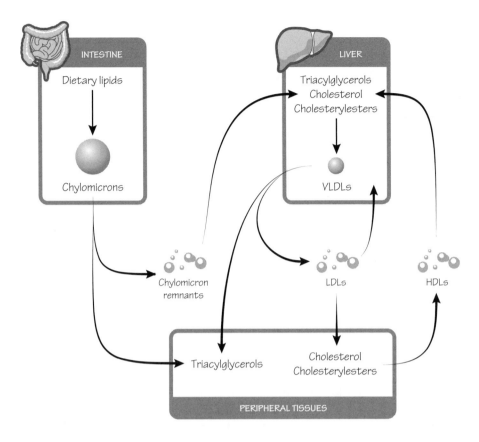

Figure 4-5 Lipid transport and metabolism. Ingested lipids are absorbed by the intestines and transformed into chylomicrons (CM). Lipoprotein lipase breaks down CM into triacylglycerols, which are delivered to peripheral tissues, and into CM remnants, which are then transported to the liver where they are endocytosed. Endogenous triacylglycerols, cholesterol, and cholesteryl esters are assembled into VLDL in the liver. As VLDLs are depleted of triglycerides by peripheral tissues, they become LDLs, which are composed mainly of cholesterol and cholesteryl esters. LDLs deliver their contents to peripheral tissue and back to the liver. Finally, HDL functions to remove excess cholesterol and cholesteryl esters from the blood and returns them to the liver.

depletes CMs of their lipoproteins. After their TGs are depleted peripherally, CMs (now called a CM remnant) are ultimately filtered, endocytosed, and removed from circulation by the liver.

- **Very low-density lipoproteins (VLDLs)**: VLDLs are produced endogenously in the liver and are primarily composed of TGs. These lipoproteins deliver lipids, made by the liver, to peripheral tissues for cellular use. As VLDLs circulate in the vascular system, lipoprotein lipase degrades the TGs of VLDLs, converting them to LDLs.

- **Low-density lipoproteins (LDLs)**: LDLs are derived from TG-depleted VLDLs. The primary role of LDL is to supply cholesterol to peripheral tissues. Thus, LDLs are composed primarily of cholesterol and cholesterol esters. Excess LDL can be problematic, since peripheral tissues do not take it up. Macrophages, which are unable to regulate their intracellular cholesterol levels, take up the excess LDL, and, over time, this accumulation of cholesterol within macrophages results in the transformation of these cells into "foam" cells. Foam cells play an integral role in the formation of atherosclerotic plaques. The use of drugs to lower serum concentrations of LDL cholesterol can reduce the progression of plaque formation, and may lead to regression of a plaque, improving circulation and ultimately reducing mortality.

- **High-density lipoproteins (HDLs)**: HDLs are lipoproteins synthesized in the liver that activate peripheral lipoprotein lipase enzymes and act to remove free cholesterol from the peripheral tissues. HDLs carry excess cholesterol back to the liver, where the HDL is degraded and the returned cholesterol is released.

Arrhythmias

Normal Conduction Pathway of the Heart

The physiologic drive of normal cardiac muscle contraction originates from specialized cells located in the sinoatrial (SA) node that are capable of spontaneous generation of action potentials. While most myocardial tissue is capable of spontaneously depolarizing, the cells of the SA node normally depolarize at the highest rate, and, therefore, serve as the pacemaker for the heart. The normal depolarization of the heart follows a conduction pathway that enables the chambers of the heart to contract efficiently. This pathway originates in the SA node and spreads throughout both atria, allowing synchronized atrial contraction (which occurs during ventricular diastole). After depolarization of the atria, the electrical impulse is funneled through another group of cells located just distal to the atrial/ventricular junction, called the atrioventricular (AV) node. This

HARDCORE

Major risk factors for developing coronary artery disease (CAD):
- Tobacco use
- Diabetes mellitus
- Hypertension
- High LDL
- Low HDL
- Family history of CAD
- Men > 45 years old
- Women > 55 years old

HARDCORE

Remember that, although antilipid drugs can effectively control cholesterol and triglyceride levels, lifestyle modification (diet alteration/restriction along with increased exercise) is the principal strategy to reducing hyperlipidemia.

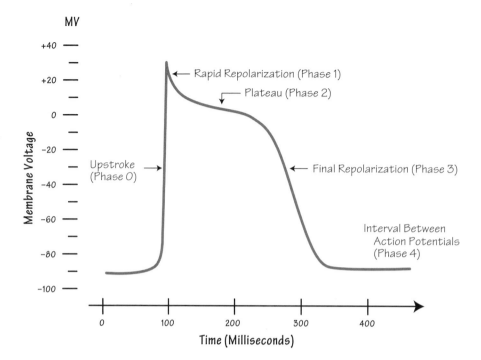

MV

Figure 4-6 A representative action potential in cardiac muscle. Phase 0 is a rapid depolarization due to Na⁺ influx following opening of Na⁺ channels. Phase 0 occurs at the same instant as the QRS complex on an electrocardiogram. Phase 1 is a rapid repolarization mediated by K⁺ efflux from the myocytes. During phase 2, membrane permeability to both Na⁺ and K⁺ is decreased, resulting in a plateau. Phase 3 is the final repolarization of the myocyte and is due to enhanced Ca^{2+} permeability across the cell membrane. Once the membrane potential has returned to its resting level between heart beats, the myocytes are in phase 4 or diastole. The action potential depicted here is characteristic of cardiac muscle tissue that does not serve as a pacemaker. Cardiac action potentials that occur in pacemaker cells differ in morphology from the action potential depicted here, with a slower upstroke mediated by Ca^{2+} influx rather than Na⁺.

group of cells, much like the cells in the SA node, has unique properties vital to cardiac conduction. AV nodal cells can serve as ventricular pacemakers in certain situations. However, normally, the pacemaking potential of the AV node is suppressed by the more rapidly depolarizing cells of the SA node. Additionally, AV node cells are unique because their action potential upstroke is not mediated by fast voltage-gated sodium channels, but rather by calcium channels that allow for slower conduction velocity between the atria and the ventricles. This decreased conduction velocity allows the atria to completely contract (atrial systole) and pump blood into the ventricles before the ventricles depolarize and contract (ventricular systole). From the AV node, conduction continues through the bundle of His, and finally spreads rapidly through the Purkinje system, resulting in ventricular contraction.

Aberrant Conduction of the Heart (Arrhythmia)

The term "*arrhythmia*" refers to a variation in the normal cardiac electrical conduction or rhythm of the heart. Arrhythmias are common clinically and may or may not represent a significant pathologic finding. There are many types of arrhythmias, including:

- **Sinus bradycardia**: Regular rhythm with a heart rate of < 60 beats per minute
- **Sinus tachycardia**: Regular rhythm with a heart rate of > 100 beats per minute
- **Atrial fibrillation (A-fib)**: In A-fib, the normal orderly activation of electrical impulses from the SA node is replaced by many rapidly firing and disorganized impulses, resulting in *chaotic contractions of the atrial muscle*. In contrast to a normal heart rate of 60 to 100 beats per minute, the rate of atrial impulses with A-fib can range from 350 to 600 beats per minute, and is very irregular. The AV node cannot conduct all of these impulses. Thus, ventricular rate rarely exceeds 170 beats per minute, and is irregular due to the irregularity of the atrial rate. A-fib is usually associated with underlying heart disease complicated by heart failure and atrial enlargement (secondary to atrial stretching that changes normal conduction), an elevation in atrial pressure, or inflammation of the atria.

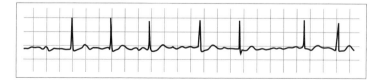

Figure 4-7(A) Atrial fibrillation. Note that P waves are irregular and wavy, ventricular rate is irregular, and QRS complex is normal. (Reprinted with permission from Axford J. Medicine. 2nd ed. Oxford: Blackwell Publishing, 2004:439.)

- **Atrial flutter**: Commonly results from a rapidly firing ectopic pacemaker site in the atria. This ectopic site can be due to the presence of a reentrant circuit or enhanced automaticity at the site. Atrial rates can be in the range of 200 to 400 beats per minute. However, not all atrial beats are conducted to the ventricles. On an ECG, atrial flutter appears as a *sawtooth pattern*, with intermittent ventricular contractions.

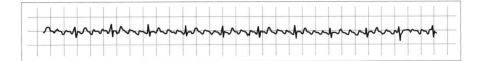

Figure 4-7(B) Atrial flutter. Note that P waves have a sawtooth pattern, QRS complex is normal, and not every P wave is conducted to the ventricles. (Reprinted with permission from Axford J. Medicine. 2nd ed. Oxford: Blackwell Publishing, 2004:439.)

- **Supraventricular tachycardia (SVT)**: This is any tachyarrhythmia that requires only atrial and/or AV nodal tissue for its initiation and maintenance. Therefore, the site of origin for SVT may be in the sinus node, the atria, the AV node, the His bundle, or some combination of these sites. SVT is commonly described as a ***narrow QRS complex tachycardia*** because conduction remains normal through the Purkinje fibers and the ventricles. Atrial tachyarrhythmias can include: sinus tachycardia, sinus nodal reentrant tachycardia, atrial tachycardia, atrial flutter, and atrial fibrillation. AV nodal tachyarrhythmias can include AV nodal reentrant tachycardia, junctional ectopic tachycardia, and nonparoxysmal junctional tachycardia.

- **Reentrant tachycardia**: Refers to the continuous, repetitive propagation of an excitatory wave traveling in a circular path within myocardial tissue (can be atrial, junctional, or ventricular) and returning to its site of origin to ***reactivate*** that site. Susceptible patients usually have an anatomic abnormality that causes changes in the heart's electrical conduction pathway, thus placing them at risk for developing reentrant tachycardia following myocardial insult (e.g., ischemia, electrolyte or pH abnormalities, or the premature cardiac contraction).

- **Ventricular tachycardia (V-tach)**: V-tach is a ***wide QRS complex tachycardia*** that originates from either a ventricular focus (no regular P waves) or from a supraventricular focus that depolarizes the ventricles via an aberrant pathway. Ventricular rates are typically in the range of 140 to 250 beats per minute. V-tach is considered a medical emergency, because very high ventricular rates can compromise cardiac output and it can rapidly evolve into ventricular fibrillation.

- **Ventricular fibrillation (V-fib)**: In V-fib, the ventricles do not beat in an organized fashion, resulting in greatly decreased cardiac output. The ECG tracing is characterized by an irregular, wavy baseline without P waves and QRS complexes. V-fib can occur following an MI, drug insult, or run of V-tach. During V-fib, the ventricles are said to resemble a "**bag of worms**," writhing with many tiny contractions, but the ***ventricles do not produce enough force to pump any blood***. V-fib is a medical emergency and requires immediate electrical defibrillation.

- **Torsades de pointes**: Torsades de pointes is a polymorphic ventricular tachycardia associated with conditions that ***prolong the QT interval***. In a patient with torsades de pointes, the peaks of the QRS complexes appear to "twist" around the isoelectric line of the recording. "Torsades de pointes" literally means "twisting of the points." Torsades de pointes can induce syncope or progress to V-fib.

HARDCORE

Although atrial flutter and atrial fibrillation change the rate of atrial tissue and often result in supraventricular tachycardia, they may not always change ventricular rate, due to the regulation of impulse conduction to the ventricles by the AV node.

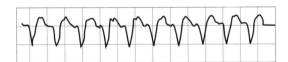

Figure 4-8(A) Ventricular tachycardia. Note P waves are not present or obscured, wide ARS complex, and ventricular rate of 140–250 bpm. (Reprinted with permission from Axford J. Medicine. 2nd ed. Oxford: Blackwell Publishing, 2004:444.)

(a) Coarse

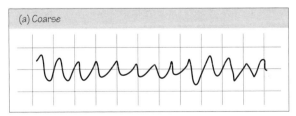

(b) Fine

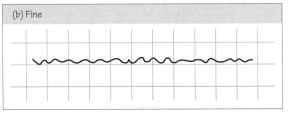

Figure 4-8(B) Ventricular fibrillation. Note chaotic, irregular pattern and no discernable P waves or QRS complexes. (Reprinted with permission from Axford J. Medicine. 2nd ed. Oxford: Blackwell Publishing, 2004:445.)

Drugs used for the treatment of arrhythmias are divided into five classes on the basis of mechanism of action.

DRUGS USED TO TREAT CARDIOVASCULAR DISEASES

There are many classes of drugs that are used in the treatment of the cardiovascular disorders described above. For the USMLE Step 1 exam you will be expected to be familiar with the following classes:

- Diuretics
- Sympatholytics
- Antiarrhythmics
- Angiotensin antagonists
- Direct-acting vasodilators
- Calcium channel antagonists
- Drugs used to treat lipid disorders

Diuretics

Diuresis refers to an increase in urine volume. Thus, a **diuretic** is an agent that promotes the production of urine. Diuretics are traditionally used in the treatment of hypertension and as an adjunct therapy to reduce edema in diseases such as congestive heart failure. Diuretics can be

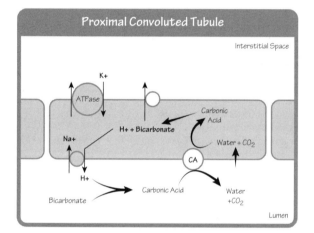

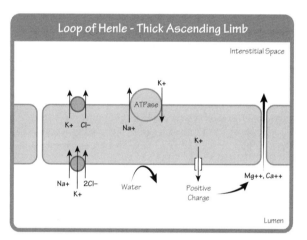

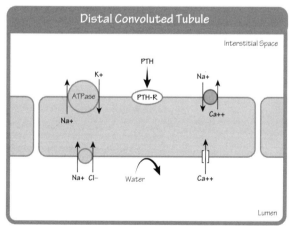

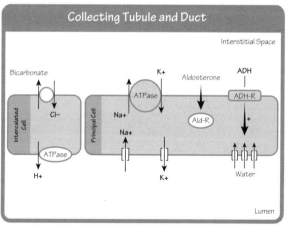

Figure 4-9 Solute reabsorption in the renal tubules. All segments possess a basolateral Na^+-K^+ ATPase, which functions to maintain the K^+ and Na^+ ionic gradients. In the **proximal convoluted tubule**, bicarbonate is converted to water and carbon dioxide (CO_2) by the enzyme carbonic anhydrase (CA). Water and CO_2 then diffuse into the cell, where they are converted back to bicarbonate and a hydrogen ion. Bicarbonate is removed by a basolateral transporter, and hydrogen ions are removed by the N^+-H^+ exhanger in order to maintain the concentration gradient necessary for bicarbonate reabsorption. The **thick ascending limb of the loop of Henle** is impermeable to water, but reabsorbs Na^+, K^+, and Cl^- ions via the Na^+/K^+/$2Cl^-$ cotransporter. Magnesium (Mg^{2+}) and calcium (Ca^{2+}) reabsorption in this segment is driven by a slight positive luminal charge that exists due to K^+ efflux. The **distal convoluted tubule** reabsorbs Na^+ and Cl^- via a Na^+/Cl^- cotransporter and is also impermeable to water. Parathyroid hormone (PTH) acts in the segment to stimulate calcium (Ca^{2+}) reabsorption by binding to receptors on the basolateral membrane. In the principal cells of the **collecting duct and tubule**, Na^+ is reabsorbed passively through Na^+ channels, which drives K^+ efflux from the cells. Aldosterone and ADH both act in this segment. The intercalated cells are responsible for acidification and alkalinization of urine.

subdivided according to the segment of the nephron in which they work. The nephron can be divided into the following segments:

A. Proximal tubule

B. Thin descending limb of the loop of Henle

C. Thick ascending limb of the loop of Henle

D. Distal convoluted tubule

E. Collecting tubule and duct

Proximal Convoluted Tubule

- 85% of the filtered $NaHCO_3$ and 40% of the filtered NaCl are reabsorbed through the action of *carbonic anhydrase*.
- 60% of filtered H_2O is passively reabsorbed.

Descending Limb of the Loop of Henle

- No solute reabsorption takes place in this segment.
- *Water is passively reabsorbed* due to the hyperosmolarity of medullary interstitium.

Ascending Limb of the Loop of Henle

- Absorbs 35% of filtered Na^+ via the *$Na^+/K^+/2Cl^-$ cotransporter* on the luminal surface
- A slightly positive luminal charge in the tubules drives the **reabsorption of Ca^{2+} and Mg^{2+} ions**.
- This region is *impermeable to water*, resulting in dilution of the luminal fluid as solute is reabsorbed; thus, the thick ascending limb of the loop of Henle is sometimes referred to as the *diluting segment*.

Distal Convoluted Tubule

- Reabsorbs about 10% of filtered Na^+ via a Na^+/Cl^- cotransporter
- This segment is also *impermeable to water*.
- Parathyroid hormone (PTH) acts in this segment to increase calcium reabsorption via apical calcium channels and basolateral $2Na^+/Ca^{2+}$ exchangers.

Collecting Tubule and Duct

- Normally reabsorbs 5% of filtered Na^+. It is the last site for the reabsorption of Na^+ ions, and, therefore, it determines the final concentration of Na^+ in the urine.
- The **principal cells** of the collecting ducts contain separate Na^+ and K^+ channels. Na^+ ions move into the principal cells due to the electrochemical forces present, resulting in a slight negative charge in the lumen. This negative charge has two effects: (1) it drives Cl^- reabsorption; and (2) it drives K^+ ion efflux from the principal cells via apical K^+ channels. Thus, the *amount of Na^+ delivered to and reabsorbed in the collecting ducts is proportional to the amount of K^+ excreted in the urine*. This loss of K^+ is known as "potassium wasting."
- **Aldosterone**, whose secretion is stimulated by angiotensin II, acts at receptors in the collecting duct to increase the transcription of Na^+ and K^+ channels, resulting in an increase in their numbers. This results in increased Na^+ reabsorption and increased K^+ wasting.
- **Antidiuretic hormone (ADH; vasopressin)** increases water permeability at the renal tubule, resulting in decreased urine volume and increased osmolality.

Carbonic Anhydrase Inhibitors

 Acetazolamide, dichlorphenamide

Indications—Glaucoma typically; metabolic alkalosis

Mechanism of Action—***Reversibly inhibits the enzyme carbonic anhydrase***. In the eye, this results in a reduction in the amount of bicarbonate secreted into the aqueous humor and a decrease in intraocular pressure. In the kidneys, inhibition of carbonic anhydrase results in a reduction in the amount of bicarbonate reabsorbed in the proximal tubule.

Side Effects—Myopia, flushing, tinnitus

Loop Diuretics

 Furosemide, ethacrynic acid, bumetanide

Loop diuretics are the most potent diuretics available.

Indications—Hypertension, edema, management of acute renal or hepatic failure, congestive heart failure

Mechanism of Action—***Inhibits the $Na^+/K^+/2Cl^-$ transporter in the thick ascending limb of the loop of Henle***

HARDCORE

Acetazolamide is contraindicated in patients with sulfa allergies.

HARDCORE

Loop diuretics are filtered by the kidney and act in the lumen of the loop of Henle. In patients with reduced glomerular filtration rates, it is not uncommon to administer large amounts of loop diuretics to achieve a level of drug within the nephron that provides the desired diuresis.

HARDCORE

Furosemide and *hydrochlorothiazide* contain sulfa in their molecular structure, and therefore are contraindicated in patients with sulfa allergies.

HARDCORE

Spironolactone is often administered together with a loop or thiazide diuretic to limit the potassium wasting associated with these agents.

HARDCORE

Reducing vascular sympathetic tone results in *decreased peripheral vascular resistance*, but also induces a baroreceptor-mediated *reflex tachycardia* that can result in myocardial ischemia in cardiac-compromised patients.

HARDCORE

α-Adrenergic receptor blockers may be associated with a "*first-dose effect*," which refers to an exaggerated hypotensive response resulting in syncope after the first dose. Therefore, it is suggested that the first dose be taken before going to bed.

HARDCORE

Pheochromocytomas are catecholamine-secreting tumors that can cause a hypertensive crisis if manipulated excessively during surgical removal. Administering *phenoxybenzamine* preoperatively prevents the excessive catecholamines released during the procedure from inducing a hypertensive crisis from systemic α-adrenergic receptor activation. A β-adrenergic receptor blocker, such as *propranolol*, is also given preoperatively.

HARDCORE

Nonselective α-adrenergic receptor blockers can cause tachycardia by two mechanisms:

- Inhibition of α_2 receptor-mediated negative feedback, resulting in increased pre-synaptic storage and release of norepinephrine (NE). The increased release of NE acts on β-adrenergic receptors and can cause a dangerous tachycardia.
- Blocking peripheral vasoconstriction leads to a reflex increase in heart rate.

Antagonists selective for α_1 receptors (*prazosin*, *terazosin*, *doxazosin*) allow α_2 receptor-mediated regulation of NE release and do not produce the same degree of tachycardia as nonselective α-adrenergic receptor blockers.

Side Effects—Orthostatic hypotension, hyperuricemia, hypokalemia ("potassium wasting"), hypomagnesemia, metabolic alkalosis, hypernatremia

Thiazide Diuretics

 Hydrochlorothiazide, hydroflumethiazide, methyclothiazide

The "-**thiazides**."

Indications—Hypertension, edema in CHF, and nephrotic syndrome

Mechanism of Action—***Inhibits NaCl reabsorption*** from the luminal surface of the distal tubule

Side Effects—Hypokalemia ("potassium wasting"), hypercalcemia, orthostatic hypotension

Potassium-Sparing Diuretics

 Spironolactone, amiloride

These agents inhibit sodium reabsorption in the late distal tubule and collecting ducts. Recall that in this segment, intracellular potassium is exchanged for intraluminal sodium. The amount of sodium reabsorbed in the collecting duct determines the amount of potassium that is excreted. Therefore, ***by preventing sodium reabsorption, potassium wasting is decreased***.

Spironolactone

Indications—Hypertension, CHF, hypokalemia

Mechanism of Action—***Antagonizes aldosterone receptors*** and prevents the translocation of the receptor complex to the nucleus. Recall that aldosterone is a steroid that increases the number of Na^+ and K^+ channels on the luminal membrane by enhancing DNA transcription of these proteins. Therefore, *spironolactone* inhibits aldosterone-mediated Na^+ reabsorption.

Side Effects—Mental confusion, agranulocytosis, hyperkalemia

Amiloride

Indications—Hypertension, edema associated with CHF, hypokalemia

Mechanism of Action—Prevents Na^+ reabsorption in the collecting ducts by blocking the Na^+ flux through luminal ion channels

Side Effects—Hyperkalemia

Sympatholytics

Sympatholytics are drugs that antagonize the sympathetic nervous system. These drugs are widely used in the treatment of cardiovascular disorders.

Adrenergic antagonists have an affinity for adrenergic receptors, but do not possess intrinsic activity at those receptors, effectively blocking endogenous activity at the receptor.

α-Adrenergic Receptor Blockers

 Prazosin, terazosin, doxazosin, phenoxybenzamine, phentolamine, yohimbine

α-Adrenergic receptors are most commonly used to lower blood pressure, since α_1 adrenergic receptors play a significant role in modulating vascular tone.

Prazosin, Terazosin, Doxazosin

Indications—Hypertension, benign prostatic hypertrophy (BPH)

Mechanism of Action—***Selective antagonists at the α_1 adrenergic receptor***, resulting in relaxation of both arterial and venous smooth muscle and decreased peripheral vascular resistance. α_1 adrenergic receptors are also found on smooth muscle fibers in the bladder neck and prostate, resulting in decreased smooth muscle tone and improved urine flow in patients with BPH.

Side Effects—Fatigue, nasal congestion, orthostatic hypotension, impotence

Phenoxybenzamine

Indications—Pheochromocytoma

Mechanism of Action—***Irreversible***, noncompetitive α_1- and α_2-adrenergic receptor antagonism

Side Effects—Postural hypotension, reflex tachycardia, angina pectoris

Phentolamine

Indications—Pheochromocytoma

Mechanism of Action—***Reversibly*** and competitively blocks both α_1- and α_2-adrenergic receptors

Side Effects—Arrhythmias, reflex tachycardia, angina pectoris, orthostatic hypotension, impotence

YOHIMBINE

Indications—Impotence (controversial)

Mechanism of Action—Blocks α_2-adrenergic receptors and **inhibits negative feedback inhibition of catecholamine release from presynaptic neurons**. This results in increased production and release of neurotransmitters from the presynaptic neuron.

Side Effects—Tachycardia, tremor

β-Adrenergic Receptor Blockers

 Propranolol, timolol, nadolol, metoprolol, atenolol, esmolol, acebutolol, pindolol

Drugs in this class block β-adrenergic receptor activation. These drugs are commonly used to lower blood pressure, but can also be employed to control heart rate, treat angina, and eliminate cardiac arrhythmias.

PROPRANOLOL

Indications

- **Hypertension**—Lowers blood pressure by decreasing cardiac output
- **Angina pectoris**—Decreases oxygen demand of the myocardium by slowing heart rate and diminishing contractility, lowering oxygen requirements
- **Myocardial infarction**—Reduces infarct size and improves recovery by blocking the effects of circulating catecholamines released due to stress
- **Congestive heart failure**—When given to a patient with stable CHF, blocking β-receptors allows the myocardium to remodel, limits stress by preventing myotoxicity caused by chronic high concentrations of catecholamines, and improves contractility by resensitizing β_1 receptors.
- **Supraventricular cardiac arrhythmias**—Slows AV nodal conduction velocity
- **Hyperthyroidism**—Antagonizes sympathetic stimulation caused by excess thyroid hormone
- **Migraine**—Blocks catecholamine-induced vasodilation in the cerebral vasculature

Mechanism of Action—Blocks β_1 and β_2 receptors leading to diminished heart rate and cardiac output by slowing AV nodal conduction velocity and decreasing myocardial contractility

Side Effects—Bronchoconstriction (due to β_2 receptor blockade), bradycardia (due to β_1 receptor blockade), impotence, depression

TIMOLOL AND NADOLOL

Indications—Glaucoma; *nadolol* is longer acting, and *timolol* is more potent when compared to *propranolol*

Mechanism of Action—Nonselective β-adrenergic receptor blockade, thereby decreasing production of aqueous humor

Side Effects—Rare if used topically; systemic side effects similar to propranolol

METOPROLOL, ATENOLOL, ESMOLOL

Indications—Hypertension, arrhythmias, angina

Mechanism of Action—Selective antagonism of β_1-adrenergic receptors located on the myocardium

Side Effects—Arrhythmias, sexual dysfunction, depression

ACEBUTOLOL AND PINDOLOL

Indications—Hypertension with moderate bradycardia

Mechanism of Action—These compounds are examples of partial agonists that appear to be antagonists. They weakly stimulate β_1- and β_2-adrenergic receptors, but have less intrinsic activity than the endogenous catecholamines, resulting in diminished heart rate and cardiac output.

Side Effects—Similar to *propranolol*

Combined α- and β-Adrenergic Receptor Blockers

This class of drugs is used for acute hypertension and tachycardia in hospital settings.

LABETALOL

Indications—Acute hypertension in which increased vascular resistance is undesirable; tachyarrhythmia; pregnancy-induced hypertension

Mechanism of Action—Reversibly blocks α_1, β_1, and β_2 receptors, resulting in decreased heart rate, cardiac output, and peripheral resistance

Side Effects—Similar to *propranolol*; also orthostatic hypotension and dizziness

HARDCORE

Never give a nonselective β-blocker (e.g., *propranolol*) to a person with asthma or COPD. Blockade of β_2-adrenergic receptors in the bronchioles can precipitate severe bronchoconstriction.

HARDCORE

Caution must be used with β-blockers in diabetics, since these drugs inhibit glucagon secretion from pancreatic islet cells and attenuate the normal physiologic response to hypoglycemia.

HARDCORE

Esmolol has a very short half-life and acts rapidly, so it is used in situations that require brief, rapid blockade (e.g., for thyroid storm).

HARDCORE

Although β-adrenergic receptor blockers are considered first line for treatment of chronic angina, certain β-blockers (especially *acebutolol* and *pindolol*) are not recommended for patients with angina, since these drugs also have intrinsic sympathomimetic activity and may exacerbate the complications of angina in some patients.

HARDCORE

By decreasing heart rate and cardiac output, other β-blockers cause a reflex increase in peripheral vascular resistance. *Labetalol*, by blocking α_1 receptors, inhibits this reflex vasoconstriction.

Modulators of Neurotransmitter Release

These drugs act within the presynaptic neuron to limit the release of neurotransmitters from storage vesicles. These agents are rarely used today (except in USMLE Step 1 questions) due to their significant side effects.

RESERPINE

Indications—Hypertension (rarely)

Mechanism of Action—*Reserpine **blocks the transport of amines from neuronal cytoplasm into storage vesicles***, allowing monoamine oxidase (MAO) in the cytoplasm to degrade excess catecholamines. This results in depletion of neurotransmitters in the nerve terminal.

Side Effects—Hypotension, bradycardia, syncope

GUANETHIDINE

Indications—Hypertension (rarely)

Mechanism of Action—Guanethidine ***blocks the storage and vesicular release of catecholamines*** from presynaptic nerve terminals.

Side Effects—Orthostatic hypotension, impotence, bradycardia

Antiarrhythmics

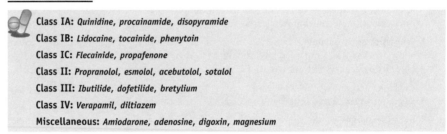

Class IA: *Quinidine, procainamide, disopyramide*
Class IB: *Lidocaine, tocainide, phenytoin*
Class IC: *Flecainide, propafenone*
Class II: *Propranolol, esmolol, acebutolol, sotalol*
Class III: *Ibutilide, dofetilide, bretylium*
Class IV: *Verapamil, diltiazem*
Miscellaneous: *Amiodarone, adenosine, digoxin, magnesium*

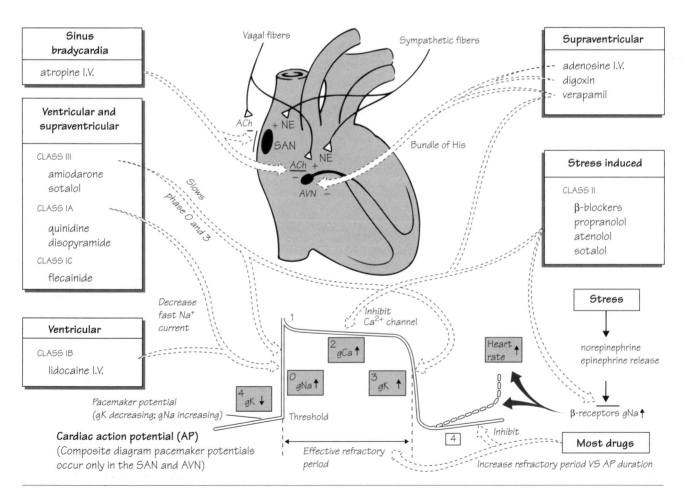

Figure 4-10 Antiarrhythmic drugs. (Reprinted with permission from Neal MJ. Medical Pharmacology at a Glance. 4th ed. Oxford: Blackwell Publishing, 2002:40.)

These drugs act by altering ion flow within the myocardium. The three ions affected by antiarrhythmics are Na^+, Ca^{2+}, and K^+. Antiarrhythmic drugs can be classified by their ability to directly or indirectly block the flux of one or more of these ions across the membranes of excitable cardiac muscle cells.

Class I: Na^+ Channel Blockers

These blockers are subdivided into ***three classes (IA, IB, IC)*** on the basis of their ability to block Na^+ channels and on their effects on the repolarization of the cardiac membrane. Remember that sodium channels are responsible for the ***initial rapid depolarization (phase 0)*** of atrial, Purkinje, and ventricular cells. Blocking Na^+ channels:

- Slows the rate and amplitude of phase 0 depolarization
- Reduces cell excitability
- Reduces conduction velocity

CLASS IA: Na^+ CHANNEL BLOCKERS

 Quinidine, procainamide, disopyramide

Indications—Supraventricular tachycardia, including atrial fibrillation/flutter, ventricular arrhythmias (premature ventricular contractions, ventricular tachycardias)

Mechanism of Action—Depresses phase 0 of the myocyte action potential and decreases myocardial excitability, conduction velocity, and contractility by ***decreasing Na^+ influx during depolarization and potassium efflux in repolarization***

Side Effects—***Prolongation of the QT interval***, which increases the risk for developing torsades de pointes

- **Procainamide**: Agranulocytosis and lupus-like syndrome
- **Quinidine**: Thrombocytopenia and cinchonism
- **Disopyramide**: Anticholinergic side effects (e.g., urinary retention)

CLASS IB: Na^+ CHANNEL BLOCKERS

 Lidocaine, tocainide, phenytoin

Indications—Used only for ventricular arrhythmias. *Lidocaine* is particularly useful for sustained ventricular tachycardia.

Mechanism of Action—Binds and blocks Na^+ channels, thereby suppressing automaticity of conduction tissue by increasing the electrical stimulation threshold of the ventricle and His-Purkinje system

Side Effects—Paresthesia, dizziness, drowsiness

CLASS IC: Na^+ CHANNEL BLOCKERS

 Flecainide, propafenone

Indications—Wolff-Parkinson-White syndrome, AV-nodal reentry arrhythmias, atrial fibrillation/flutter

Mechanism of Action—Very high potency Na^+ channel blocker that markedly decreases speed of conduction but with no effect on repolarization

Side Effects—As a class, they all may cause dizziness and nausea, and similar to all other antiarrhythmics they can be ***proarrhythmic***.

Class II: β-Adrenergic Receptor Blockers

 Propranolol, esmolol, acebutolol, sotalol

Indications—Paroxysmal supraventricular tachycardia, control of ventricular rate in atrial fibrillation/flutter, suppression of premature ventricular tachycardia

Mechanism of Action—Blocks β-adrenergic receptors, which results in decreased Ca^{2+} influx in the AV and SA nodes. This results in ***a slow sinus rhythm and a prolonged PR interval***. These drugs do not have any effect on the QRS or QT intervals.

Hardcore—*Sotalol* is the exception, in that in addition to acting as a β-blocker, it can ***prolong QT interval by blockage of K^+ channels*** (class III effect).

Side Effects—Heart block, hypotension, heart failure, bronchospasm, fatigue, impotence

Class III: K^+ Channel Blockers

 Ibutilide, dofetilide, bretylium

HARDCORE

Procainamide is acetylated by the liver to form the active ***metabolite N-acetylprocainamide (NAPA)***, which is cleared by the kidneys. Care should be taken when using this drug in patients with renal impairment.

HARDCORE

Cinchonism is a syndrome characterized by nausea/vomiting, diarrhea, and CNS effects including tinnitus, vertigo, headache, and auditory/visual disturbances.

HARDCORE

Sotalol is useful for treatment and prevention of atrial fibrillation.

Indications—Atrial fibrillation/flutter

Mechanism of Action—Blocks outward potassium channels, leading to prolonged repolarization (i.e., *prolongs QT interval and increases refractoriness*). These drugs have little to no effect on depolarization (i.e., QRS interval).

Side Effects—Hypotension, torsades de pointes

Class IV: Ca²⁺ Channel Blockers

 Verapamil, diltiazem

Indications—Supraventricular tachycardias including atrial fibrillation/flutter, atrial automaticities, AV nodal reentry

Mechanism of Action—Selectively *blocks AV nodal L-type calcium channels*, leading to a slow sinus rhythm and a prolonged PR interval (i.e., increases AV-node refractoriness), with no effect on QRS interval. Ca²⁺ channel blockade also leads to decreased contractility.

Side Effects—Hypotension, sinus bradycardia, constipation

Miscellaneous

 Amiodarone, adenosine, digoxin, magnesium

This is a collection of drugs that act by distinct mechanisms or by a combination of the above classes of antiarrhythmics.

AMIODARONE
Principally a class III agent with multiple other effects.

Indications—Ventricular tachycardia/fibrillation, to prevent sustained ventricular tachycardia/fibrillation and premature ventricular tachycardia, atrial fibrillation

Mechanism of Action—Blocks:

- Na⁺ channels (<u>class I effects</u>)
- β-adrenergic receptors (<u>class II effects</u>)
- K⁺ channels (<u>class III effects</u>)
- α-adrenergic receptors
- Muscarinic receptors

Side Effects—*Pulmonary fibrosis*, increased liver enzymes with progression to cirrhosis and fatal hepatic necrosis, hypothyroidism or hyperthyroidism, *blue-gray discoloration of skin*, corneal deposits, optic neuritis and loss of vision, peripheral neuropathy, increased LDH, torsades de pointes

ADENOSINE

Indications—*Paroxysmal supraventricular tachycardia*

Mechanism of Action—Enhances potassium conduction and inhibits cAMP-induced Ca²⁺ influx, *slowing conduction and interrupting reentrant pathways through AV node*

Side Effects—Hypotension, flushing, chest pain, and dyspnea associated with infusion; metallic taste; bronchospasm, particularly in patients with reactive airway disease and thus should be used cautiously in these patients

DIGOXIN

Indications—Paroxysmal supraventricular arrhythmias (e.g., AV nodal reentry), atrial fibrillation/flutter

Mechanism of Action—Digoxin is used for heart failure and SVT:

- **Heart failure**: Inhibits the sodium/potassium ATPase pump, which increases the intracellular Na⁺–Ca²⁺exchange to increase intracellular calcium, leading to increased contractility
- **SVT**: Directly suppresses AV node conduction, increases the effective refractory period and decreases conduction velocity including positive inotropic effects, enhances vagal tone, and decreases ventricular rate

Side Effects—Anorexia, vomiting, diarrhea, headache, confusion, abnormal vision (aura)

MAGNESIUM

Indications—Torsades de pointes and arrhythmias related to digitalis toxicity

Mechanism of Action—Unknown

Side Effects—Hypotension, ECG changes

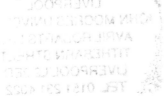

HARDCORE

β-blockers in conjunction with calcium channel blockers can lead to a complete AV-nodal block, leading to heart block.

HARDCORE

Amiodarone has a very long half-life, which can result in prolongation of its many toxicities.

HARDCORE

Adenosine has a **short half-life in blood** (< **10 seconds**), which tends to minimize side effects.

HARDCORE

An antibody that binds to *digoxin* and removes it from circulation is used to treat *digoxin* overdose.

TABLE 4-2	Indication Guide for Arrhythmias		
	TREATMENT GOALS	**FIRST LINE**	**SECOND LINE**
Atrial arrhythmias (Atrial fibrillation and flutter)	• Control rhythm (decrease HR) • Slow conduction velocity	• β-blocker (*propranolol*) • Calcium-channel blocker (*diltiazem, verapamil*) • Anticoagulation	• *Quinidine* • *Amiodarone* • *Digoxin*
Supraventricular tachycardia (PSVT, AV node reentry and narrow complex)	• Slow AV node conduction velocity	• β-blocker (*propranolol*) • Calcium-channel blocker (*diltiazem, verapamil*) • *Adenosine* (PSVT)	• *Digoxin*
Ventricular arrhythmias (V-tach/V-fib)	• Slow HR • Restore normal conduction pathway • Inhibit onset of V-fib	• *Lidocaine*	• *Sotalol* • *Amiodarone* • *Bretylium*

TABLE 4-3	Major Side Effects Associated with Each Class of Antiarrhythmic		
CLASS I	**CLASS II**	**CLASS III**	**CLASS IV**
Negative inotropism	Sinus bradycardia	Sinus bradycardia	Sinus bradycardia
IA: Torsades de pointes	AV block	Torsades de pointes	AV block
IC: Monomorphic sustained V-tach	↓ Left ventricular function		Negative inotropism

Angiotensin Antagonists

Angiotensin II is a peptide produced by the enzyme angiotensin-converting enzyme (ACE) within the pulmonary system from angiotensin I (Figure 4-11). Angiotensin II increases blood pressure by (1) vasoconstriction and increasing total peripheral resistance, and (2) increasing Na^+ and water retention by stimulating aldosterone secretion. The AT-1 receptor mediates cardiovascular and adrenal gland responses to angiotensin II.

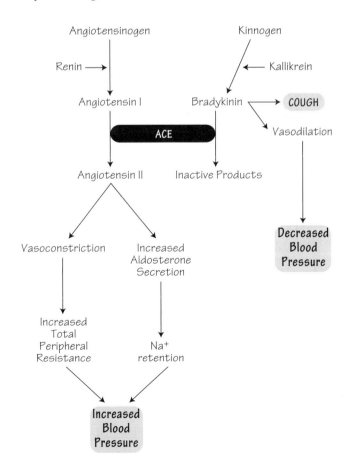

Figure 4-11 The renin-angiotensin system. The precursor peptide angiotensinogen is converted to angiotensin I by renin. Angiotensin-converting enzyme (ACE) then converts the inactive angiotensin I into active angiotensin II. Angiotensin II acts in a number of ways to increase blood pressure. ACE is also responsible for the breakdown of bradykinin. Since bradykinin is a potent vasodilator, the breakdown of bradykinin by ACE indirectly results in an increase in blood pressure.

HARDCORE

Blockade of angiotensin II formation results in the loss of the negative feedback of angiotensin II on renin secretion. Thus, plasma renin levels may be increased following administration of an ACE inhibitor.

HARDCORE

Blockade of the AT-1 receptor by ARBS also inhibits the negative feedback of angiotensin II on renin secretion, resulting in an increase in plasma renin levels. However, this increased renin activity is not sufficient to overcome the blood pressure-lowering effect of blockade of the AT-1 receptor.

HARDCORE

Use of drugs that act on the renin-angiotensin system has been associated with fetal and neonatal injury, including renal failure and oligohydramnios (not enough amniotic fluid). Thus, ACE inhibitors and ARBs should not be used in women who are pregnant, or plan to become pregnant.

HARDCORE

Nitroglycerin is administered sublingually because it undergoes extensive first-pass metabolism when given orally. Sublingual administration also results in a rapid onset of action.

HARDCORE

Isosorbide dinitrate can be administered orally, since it does not undergo extensive first-pass metabolism. *Isosorbide dinitrate* also has a longer half-life than nitroglycerin, but is not as potent.

HARDCORE

The *minoxidil* stimulation of hair growth is secondary to vasodilation, increased cutaneous blood flow, and stimulation of resting hair follicles.

HARDCORE

Administration of hydralazine and minoxidil results in a significant drop in blood pressure and a *reflex tachycardia*. This tachycardia increases myocardial oxygen demand and may result in angina pectoris, myocardial infarction, or heart failure in susceptible patients. In addition, aldosterone levels and Na+ retention are increased secondary to an increase in renin levels. Thus, these agents are given in combination with a β-blocker and a diuretic to counter these effects.

HARDCORE

Sodium nitroprusside is metabolized rapidly and therefore must be administered continuously by intravenous infusion.

HARDCORE

Sodium nitroprusside can be toxic in high doses (especially orally), because its metabolism produces *cyanide*.

There are two major classes of angiotensin antagonists used clinically:
- ACE inhibitors—prevent the conversion of angiotensin I to angiotensin II
- Angiotensin receptor blockers (ARBs)—antagonize angiotensin II at its receptor

ACE Inhibitors

Quinapril, captopril, ramipril, lisinopril, trandolapril

The "**-pril**" drugs.

Indications—Hypertension, heart failure, renal protection in diabetics

Mechanism of Action—***Prevents the formation of angiotensin II and the breakdown of bradykinin by inhibiting ACE***, resulting in a decrease in total peripheral resistance and an increase in cardiac output. Aldosterone-stimulated Na+ retention is also inhibited since aldosterone release is stimulated by angiotensin II.

Side Effects—***Cough*** and angioedema due to buildup of bradykinin

ARBs

Losartan, candesartan, irbesartan, valsartan, telmisartan

The "**-sartan**" drugs.

Indications—Hypertension; in patients with adverse reactions to ACE inhibitors

Mechanism of Action—Selective ***blockade of the binding of angiotensin II to the AT-1 receptor***

Side Effects—Hypotension, dizziness, insomnia

Vasodilators

Nitrates: *Nitroglycerin, isosorbide dinitrate*
Direct-acting smooth muscle relaxants: *Hydralazine, minoxidil, sodium nitroprusside*
Calcium channel antagonists: *Nifedipine, verapamil, diltiazem, felodipine, nisoldipine*

Nitrates

Nitroglycerin, isosorbide dinitrate

Indications—Angina pectoris, heart failure

Mechanism of Action—Nitrates ***increase nitric oxide (NO)***, a potent vasodilator. NO relaxes coronary blood vessels, resulting in an increase in blood flow and oxygen supply to the myocardium. NO also dilates the venous system, resulting in an increase in venous capacitance, and a decrease in preload on the heart, resulting in a decrease in myocardial oxygen demand.

Side Effects—***Severe headache, reflex tachycardia***

Direct-Acting Smooth Muscle Relaxants

Hydralazine, minoxidil, sodium nitroprusside

Direct-acting vasodilators are agents that act directly on vascular smooth muscle, resulting in vasodilatation. These agents are employed for both the treatment of hypertension and during hypertensive crises.

HYDRALAZINE AND MINOXIDIL

Indications—Hypertension (rarely), pre-eclampsia/eclampsia, primary pulmonary hypertension; hair loss (*minoxidil* only)

Mechanism of Action—Directly ***relaxes arteriolar smooth muscle***, with little effect on veins, effects may be mediated by cAMP

Side Effects—Reflex tachycardia; sodium and water retention; ***lupus-like syndrome (hydralazine only)***

SODIUM NITROPRUSSIDE

Indications—Hypertensive crisis (diastolic blood pressure > 130 mm Hg)

Mechanism of Action—***Releases NO***, resulting in rapid vasodilatation and a decrease in blood pressure

Side Effects—Reflex tachycardia

Calcium Channel Antagonists

Nifedipine, verapamil, diltiazem, felodipine, nisoldipine

NIFEDIPINE

Indications—Stable angina, hypertension

Mechanism of Action—Inhibits calcium ion influx into vascular smooth muscle and the myocardium, resulting in relaxation of vascular smooth muscle and vasodilatation. *Myocardial oxygen supply is enhanced* due to coronary vasodilatation.

Side Effects—Palpitations, peripheral edema, flushing

VERAPAMIL AND DILTIAZEM

Indications—Variant angina, angina pectoris, hypertension, arrhythmias (PSVT, atrial fibrillation, and atrial flutter)

Mechanism of Action—Blocks myocardial and smooth muscle calcium channels, resulting in:

- *Slowing of conduction through the AV node*
- Dilation of coronary vessels, resulting in an increased oxygen supply to the heart
- Inhibition of coronary artery vasospasm—important for *treatment of Prinzmetal's angina*
- Decreased afterload and systemic vascular resistance, reducing blood pressure and myocardial oxygen consumption

Side Effects—Bradycardia, AV node block, accelerated progression of CHF

FELODIPINE AND NISOLDIPINE

Indications—Hypertension, congestive heart failure

Mechanism of Action—Inhibits calcium influx into vascular smooth muscle and the myocardium, resulting in relaxation of vascular smooth muscle and vasodilation. Myocardial oxygen supply is enhanced due to coronary vasodilation

Side Effects—Headache, flushing, peripheral edema

Drugs Used to Treat Lipid Disorders

HARDCORE

Gingival hyperplasia is associated with *verapamil* use.

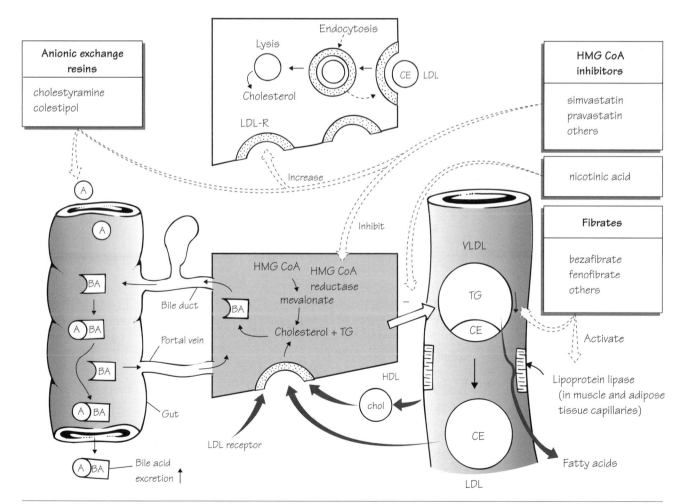

Figure 4-12 Lipid-lowering drugs. (Reprinted with permission from Neal MJ. Medical Pharmacology at a Glance. 4th ed. Oxford: Blackwell Publishing, 2002:46.)

HMG CoA Reductase Inhibitors

 Atorvastatin, fluvastatin, lovastatin, pravastatin, simvastatin

The "*-statins*."

3-Hydroxy 3-methyl **g**lutaryl-**c**oenzyme **A** reductase, or *HMG CoA reductase*, is a hepatocellular enzyme that catalyzes the rate-limiting step in cholesterol synthesis (the conversion of HMG CoA to mevalonic acid). Inhibition of HMG CoA reductase prevents the hepatic production of cholesterol, resulting in decreased hepatic cholesterol concentrations. This causes cells to increase the number of LDL receptors on their surfaces, resulting in increased uptake of circulating LDL and a drop in plasma LDL concentrations. Clinically, HMG CoA reductase inhibitors are the most effective lipid-reducing agent in lowering plasma concentrations of LDL. In addition, they have the capacity to reduce triglyceride levels and increase HDL levels.

Indications—Hyperlipidemia with elevated LDL and/or TG levels

Mechanism of Action—*Inhibition of HMG CoA reductase*

Side Effects

- GI disturbances and mild myalgias are most common.
- High doses of statins can produce *severe myalgias and muscle weakness*, and an increase in plasma creatine phosphokinase (CPK) levels can occur. This has the potential to progress to *rhabdomyolysis*, leading to *myoglobinuria* and *renal dysfunction*.
- 1% to 2% of patients on high-dose statin therapy experience elevations in liver enzymes.

Fibric Acid Derivatives (Fibrates)

 Gemfibrozil, clofibrate, fenofibrate

Indications—Hypertriglyceridemia, clinically subnormal HDL levels

Mechanism of Action—Not completely understood, but probably involves the inhibition of lipolysis, decreasing subsequent hepatic fatty acid uptake. Inhibition of hepatic secretion of VLDL may also play a role.

Side Effects

- *Myositis*
- Risk of rhabdomyolysis is *increased* if taken with statins
- Cholelithiasis (gallstones)
- Hepatitis

Nicotinic Acid

 Niacin

Indications—Hypertriglyceridemia, elevated LDL, low HDL

Mechanism of Action—*Inhibits VLDL secretion* and *suppresses VLDL synthesis*

Side Effects

- Diffuse skin flushing and pruritus
- Blurry vision
- GI distress
- Aggravation of peptic ulcers
- Hepatoxicity
- *Elevation of uric acid and blood sugar*. Care must be taken when niacin is given to patients with gout or diabetes.

Bile Acid Resins

 Cholestyramine, colestipol

Indications—Elevated LDL

Mechanism of Action—These agents *bind bile acids in the gut*, preventing the enterohepatic recirculation of bile acids. This promotes the hepatic up-regulation of 7-α-hydroxylase, and thus the conversion of cholesterol in the liver into bile acids. This promotes the up-regulation of LDL receptor expression secondary to decreased levels of cholesterol within the liver, and ultimately *leads to an enhanced removal of LDL and VLDL from the circulation*.

Side Effects—GI disturbances, including constipation, heartburn, nausea, burping, bloating, and flatulence

HARDCORE REVIEW – CARDIOVASCULAR AND RENAL PHARMACOLOGY

TABLE 4-4 Overview of Physiologic Actions for the Major Cardiovascular Drugs/Classes

	CARDIAC OUTPUT	PERIPHERAL VASCULAR RESISTANCE	AFTERLOAD	PRELOAD	MYOCARDIAL DEMAND	CORONARY VESSEL BLOOD SUPPLY
Loop and thiazide diuretics	No change	↓	↓	No change	↓	No change
α-Blockers	↑	↓	↓	↓	↓ or no change	↑
β-Blockers	↓	↓ or no change	↓ or no change	↑	↓	No change
Angiotensin antagonists	↑	↓	↓	↓	↓	No change
Hydralazine	↑	↓	↓	No change	↓ or no change	↑
Nitroglycerin	No change	↓	↓	↓	↓	↑
Diltiazem, verapamil	↓	No change	No change	↑	↓	No change

TABLE 4-5 Diuretics

DRUG CLASS	DRUGS	MECHANISM OF ACTION	MAJOR SIDE EFFECTS
Carbonic anhydrase inhibitors	*Acetazolamide, dichlorphenamide*	Reversibly inhibits carbonic anhydrase	Myopia, flushing, tinnitus
Loop diuretics	*Furosemide, ethacrynic acid, bumetanide*	Inhibits $Na^+/K^+/2Cl^-$ transporter in the thick ascending loop of Henle	Hypokalemia, hypocalcemia, metabolic alkalosis, hypernatremia
Thiazide diuretics	*Hydrochlorothiazide, hydroflumethiazide, methyclothiazide*	Inhibits NaCl reabsorption from the distal tubule	Hypokalemia, hypocalcemia
Potassium-sparing diuretics	*Spironolactone*	Antagonizes aldosterone receptors	Gynecomastia, hyperkalemia
	Amiloride	Prevents Na^+ reabsorption in the collecting ducts	Hyperkalemia

TABLE 4-6 Antiarrhythmics

DRUG CLASS	DRUGS	MECHANISM OF ACTION	MAJOR SIDE EFFECTS
Class IA: Na^+-channel blockers	*Quinidine*	Decreases sodium influx during depolarization and potassium efflux in repolarization	Prolongs QT interval, thrombocytopenia, cinchonism
	Procainamide	Decreases sodium influx during depolarization and potassium efflux in repolarization	Prolongs QT interval, agranulocytosis, produces NAPA metabolite
	Disopyramide	Decreases sodium influx during depolarization and potassium efflux in repolarization	Prolongs QT interval, anticholinergic effects
Class IB: Na^+-channel blockers	*Lidocaine, tocainide, phenytoin*	Binds and blocks sodium channels	Paresthesia, dizziness
Class IC: Na^+-channel blockers	*Flecainide, propafenone*	Very high potency Na^+-channel blockers	Proarrhythmics
Class II: β-blockers	*Propranolol, esmolol, acebutolol, sotalol*	Blocks β-adrenergic receptors, decreases Ca channel influx in AV and SA node	Heart block, bronchoconstriction, hypotension
Class III: K^+-channel blockers	*Ibutilide, dofetilide, bretylium*	Prolongs QT interval and increases refractoriness	Hypotension, torsades de pointes
Class IV: Ca^{2+}-channel blockers	*Verapamil, diltiazem*	Blocks AV nodal L-type Ca^{2+} channels	Hypotension, bradycardia, AV node block
Miscellaneous	*Amiodarone*	Blocks: • Na^+ channels • β-adrenergic receptors • K^+ channels • α-adrenergic receptors • Muscarinic receptors	Pulmonary fibrosis, hepatic necrosis, hypo- or hyperthyroidism, blue-gray skin discoloration
	Adenosine	Slows conduction and interrupts reentrant pathways through AV node	Hypotension, flushing, chest pain, dyspnea
	Digoxin	Suppresses AV node conduction, enhances vagal tone, decreases ventricular rate	Vomiting, confusion, abnormal vision (aura)

TABLE 4-7 Angiotensin Antagonists

Drug Class	Drugs	Mechanism of Action	Major Side Effects
ACE inhibitors	*Quinapril, captopril, ramipril, lisinopril, trandolapril*	Prevents both the formation of angiotensin II and the breakdown of bradykinin by inhibiting ACE	Cough, angioedema
Angiotensin receptor blockers (ARBs)	*Losartan, candesartan, irbesartan, valsartan, telmisartan*	Selectively blocks the binding of Ang II to the AT-1 receptor	Hypotension, dizziness

TABLE 4-8 Vasodilators

Drug Class	Drugs	Mechanism of Action	Major Side Effects
Nitrates	*Nitroglycerin, isosorbide dinitrate*	Produces nitric oxide (NO)	Severe headache, reflex tachycardia
Direct-acting smooth muscle relaxants	*Hydralazine, minoxidil*		Reflex tachycardia
	Sodium nitroprusside	Releases NO	Reflex tachycardia, cyanide toxicity
Calcium channel antagonists	*Nifedipine*	Inhibits calcium channels	Palpitations, peripheral edema, flushing
	Verapamil, diltiazem	Inhibits calcium channels	Bradycardia, AV node block, accelerated progression of CHF
	Felodipine, nisoldipine	Inhibits calcium channels	Headache, flushing, peripheral edema

TABLE 4-9 Agents Used to Treat Lipid Disorders

Drug Class	Drugs	Mechanism of Action	Major Side Effects
HMG CoA reductase inhibitors	*Atorvastatin, fluvastatin, lovastatin, pravastatin, simvastatin*	Inhibits HMG CoA reductase	Rhabdomyolysis, myoglobinuria, renal dysfunction
Fibric acid derivates (fibrates)	*Gemfibrozil, clofibrate, fenofibrate*	Inhibit lipolysis and the hepatic secretion of VLDL	Myositis when taken with statins
Nicotinic acid	*Niacin*	Inhibits VLDL synthesis and secretion	Skin flushing, pruritis
Bile acid resins	*Cholestyramine, colestipol*	Binds bile acids in the gut	Constipation, heartburn, nausea

CHAPTER 5

Hematological Pharmacology

The process of **hemostasis** follows a traumatic injury to the vascular system, and refers to the vasoconstriction and blood clot formation at the site of injury that act to limit bleeding from a damaged vessel. Clot formation occurs following a series of interactions between clotting factors that have been released by the injured tissue, platelets, and plasma coagulation factors (Figure 5-1).

When a pathologic thrombus forms, it typically follows the same physiological steps of clot formation, except the initial stimulus of clot development results from a pathologic condition rather than a typical traumatic event.

Therapeutic intervention for patients presenting with abnormal hemodynamic conditions, particularly thrombus formation, targets three major components of clot formation and breakdown:

1. Chemomodulators of platelet action
2. The factors that make up the coagulation cascade
3. Thrombolysis of existing clots

For the board exam, it is extremely important to understand the actions and side effects of drugs affecting platelet function and hemostasis, including the nonsteroidal anti-inflammatory drugs (*NSAIDs*), the anticoagulants *heparin* and *warfarin*, and the antidotes for anticoagulation overdose.

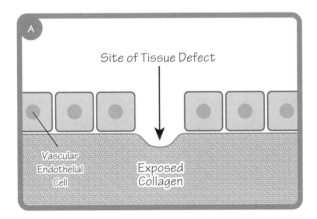
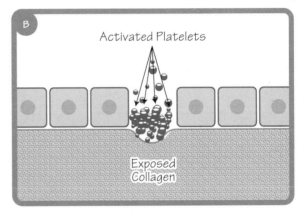
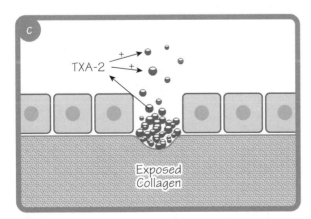
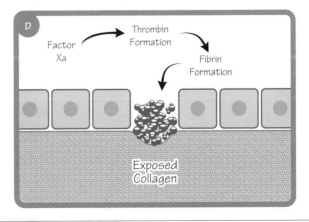

Figure 5-1 (A) Damage to the vascular endothelium exposes the underlying tissue containing collagen; **(B)** platelets from the plasma adhere to the exposed collagen; **(C)** platelets bound to collagen release thromboxane A$_2$ (TXA-2), which further promotes platelet adesion to the damaged region; **(D)** clotting Factor Xa (activation of Factor X is shown in Figure 5-3) converts prothrombin to thrombin, which in turn converts fibrinogen to fibrin. Fibrin is incorporated into the platelet plug and is cross-linked with other fibrin molecules to stabilize the clot.

PLATELET AGGREGATION INHIBITORS

 Aspirin, abciximab, dipyridamole, ticlopidine, clopidogrel

Aspirin

Indications and Usage—Pain relief, reduction of inflammation, fever reduction, anticoagulation

Mechanism of Action—The enzyme cyclooxygenase (COX) is responsible for the production of eicosanoids, including prostaglandins, from arachidonic acid (Figure 5-2). COX has several isoforms, including **COX-I and COX-II**. Both subtypes are constitutively expressed in various tissues; however, COX II is also inducible and is up-regulated during inflammation and pain. The COX-I isoform is constitutively expressed in platelets, where it is responsible for the production of the proaggregatory compound thromboxane A_2 (TXA_2). **Aspirin prevents TXA_2 formation in platelets by irreversibly inhibiting COX I.**

Side Effects—Peptic ulcer disease, **gastrointestinal bleeding**, hemorrhagic stroke, exacerbation of asthma due to bronchoconstriction

Abciximab

Indications and Usage—Prophylaxis against ischemic-cardiac events in patients undergoing percutaneous coronary interventions; given intravenously

Mechanism of Action—The glycoprotein IIb/IIIa receptor is a major platelet surface receptor involved in platelet aggregation. *Abciximab* is a **monoclonal antibody directed at the glycoprotein IIb/IIIa receptor on platelets**, and prevents the binding of fibrinogen and von Willebrand factor.

- Remember: **Ab-cixim-Ab** is an **Ab (antibody)**

Side Effects—Bleeding

Dipyridamole

Indications and Usage—Used in conjunction with *warfarin* for the prevention of embolus formation in patients with prosthetic heart valves

Mechanism of Action—**Inhibits adenosine deaminase and phosphodiesterase**, which causes an accumulation of adenosine and cyclic AMP. These mediators inhibit platelet aggregation and may cause vasodilation.

Side Effects—Bleeding

HARDCORE

Low-dose *aspirin* has been shown to decrease mortality and **reduce the incidence of thrombus-induced ischemic events**. *Aspirin* is recommended in all patients over the age of 50 and those under the age of 50 with, or at risk of, coronary artery disease (CAD).

HARDCORE

Aspirin is an irreversible, nonselective inhibitor of the COX enzyme; thus the effects of *aspirin* last the entire lifespan of the platelets. *Ibuprofen* is a reversible, nonselective inhibitor of the COX enzyme, and its effects do not span the life of a platelet.

HARDCORE

A patient who overdoses on *aspirin* can present with tinnitus, renal dysfunction, and **respiratory alkalosis** (early) with **anion gap metabolic acidosis**.

HARDCORE

The antiplatelet effects of *abciximab* last for 2 to 48 hours.

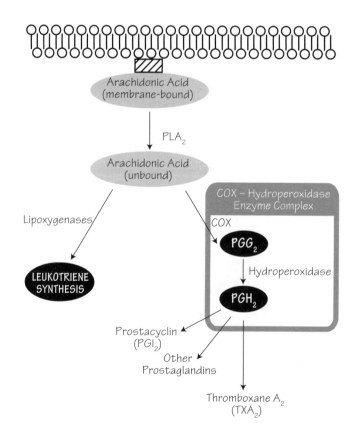

Figure 5-2 The arachidonic acid cascade.
Arachidonic acid, liberated from the membrane by phospholipase A_2 (PLA_2), can be converted to various products via several different pathways. Two of these pathways, the lipoxygenase pathway and the cyclooxygenase (COX) pathway, are depicted here. The product formed depends upon the enzymes present in a particular tissue. Aspirin and other NSAIDs are able to inhibit COX, thereby preventing prostaglandin formation.

Ticlopidine and Clopidogrel

Indications and Usage—Prophylaxis against thrombotic stroke

Mechanism of Action—Irreversibly *inhibit the ADP receptor on platelets*. Normally, stimulation of this receptor stimulates the adhesion of platelets.

Side Effects—Prolonged bleeding, *agranulocytosis*, and neutropenia

ANTICOAGULANTS

> *Heparin, warfarin, enoxaprin, dalteparin*

Two coagulation pathways are capable of thrombus formation: *the intrinsic system and extrinsic system*. Both systems involve a cascade of enzymatic reactions that activate specific proenzymes, ultimately resulting in the production of thrombin (Figure 5-3). Thrombin formation results in the generation of fibrin from fibrinogen and activates clotting factors to stabilize and cross-link fibrin molecules. Anticoagulants act on key components of this cascade to ultimately interfere with thrombus formation.

Heparin

Indications and Usage—Deep venous thrombosis (DVT; limits the expansion of thrombi), pulmonary embolism, and myocardial infarction; prevention of postoperative stasis venous thrombosis; prevention of acute thrombosis due to atrial fibrillation

Mechanism of Action—Binds *antithrombin III (ATIII)*, resulting in a conformational change that allows ATIII to rapidly *combine with and inhibit thrombin*. This prevents thrombin from converting fibrinogen to fibrin. Also binds and inhibits coagulation factor Xa.

Side Effects—Hemorrhage

HARDCORE

These agents are second line (to *aspirin*) for the prevention of thrombosis because of their serious side effects.

HARDCORE

Pregnant women can use *heparin* for anticoagulation because, unlike *warfarin*, it does not cross the placenta.

HARDCORE

Heparin is only administered parenterally and acts rapidly (within minutes).

HARDCORE

Heparin can be monitored clinically by following the *activated partial thromboplastin time (aPTT)*, a measure of the intrinsic clotting cascade.

HARDCORE

Excessive bleeding caused by *heparin* administration can be treated with *protamine sulfate*, which inactivates the heparin complex.

HARDCORE

Heparin can cause heparin-induced thrombocytopenia (HIT) or paradoxical heparin-associated thrombocytopenia thrombosis (HAT).

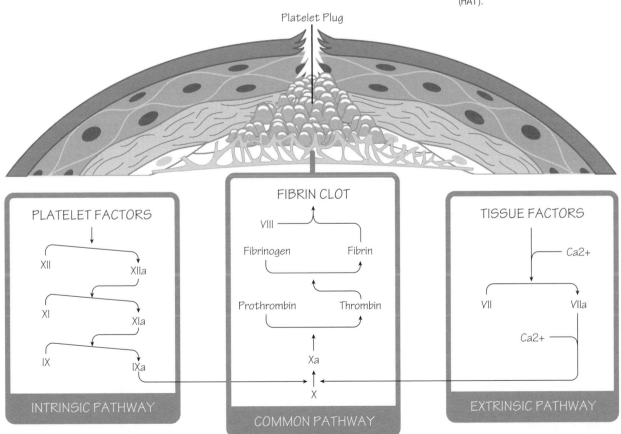

Figure 5-3 Clotting factors involved in formation of a fibrin clot. The clotting cascade contains two pathways that share a final common pathway. The extrinsic pathway is activated by factors from injured tissue. The intrinsic pathway begins with the activation of factor XII by factors released by platelets.

Enoxaparin and Dalteparin

These drugs are low molecular weight heparins.

Indications and Usage—Prophylaxis for **DVT**, especially after hip replacement; treatment of acute DVT and pulmonary embolism

Mechanism of Action—**Binds and inhibits ATIII**, causing a conformational change that allows ATIII to rapidly combine with and inhibit thrombin. This prevents thrombin from converting fibrinogen to fibrin. The *low molecular weight heparins* do not inhibit antithrombin III as potently as *heparin*.

Side Effects—Similar to *heparin*, including hemorrhage, thrombocytopenia, and osteoporosis

Warfarin

Indications and Usage—Prevention of thrombus formation (oral)

Mechanism of Action—**Clotting factors II, VII, IX, and X, and protein C and S, are dependent upon vitamin K for their synthesis in the liver.** During the synthesis of these clotting factors, vitamin K is reduced to vitamin K epoxide. The regeneration of vitamin K from vitamin K epoxide requires the enzyme vitamin K epoxide reductase. **Warfarin inhibits vitamin K epoxide reductase**, thereby preventing clotting factor *II, VII, IX, and* X formation.

Side Effects—Bleeding, headache, shortness of breath. *Warfarin* has a narrow therapeutic index, so it is essential to monitor patients who are on this drug.

THROMBOLYTICS

 Alteplase, streptokinase, urokinase

Alteplase

Alteplase is a tissue plasminogen activator (tPA) produced by recombinant DNA technology.

Indications and Usage—Myocardial infarction, acute ischemic stroke, pulmonary embolism

Mechanism of Action—Converts plasminogen bound to fibrin within a clot to plasmin, which endogenously cleaves fibrin and lyses the thrombi. **tPA binds only plasminogen already bound to fibrin**.

Side Effects—Bleeding

Streptokinase

Indications and Usage—Acute pulmonary embolism, DVT, acute myocardial infarction, occluded access shunts

Mechanism of Action—Forms an active complex with plasminogen, **converting plasminogen to plasmin, resulting in clot dissolution**. *Streptokinase* also catalyzes the degradation of fibrinogen and clotting factors V and VII.

Side Effects—Bleeding, hypersensitivity reactions including fever, rash, and **anaphylaxis**

Urokinase

Indications and Usage—Pulmonary embolism, DVT

Mechanism of Action—Directly degrades both fibrin and fibrinogen without need of binding to plasminogen first

Side Effects—Bleeding

DRUGS USED TO TREAT INFLAMMATION

Inflammation is a localized protective response elicited by injury or destruction of tissues that serves to destroy, dilute, or sequester the agent responsible for the injury as well as the injured tissue. Acute inflammation is characterized by the classic signs of pain, heat, redness, swelling, and loss of function.

Occasionally, inflammation can be inappropriately triggered in certain pathologic processes such as asthma or arthritis. Normally harmless agents such as pollen can also cause inflammation in sensitive individuals. In these situations, the inflammatory response contributes to tissue injury and requires suppression with drugs that are able to control the inflammatory response.

Although many chemical mediators contribute to the inflammatory response, the majority of anti-inflammatory drugs targets the production of prostaglandins and thromboxane. Prostaglandins and thromboxane are eicosanoids synthesized from arachidonic acid by the COX pathway (see Figure 5-2).

Nonsteroidal Anti-Inflammatory Drugs

Aspirin

Propionic acid derivatives: *Ibuprofen, fenoprofen, ketoprofen, oxaprozin*

Indoleacetic acids: *Indomethacin, sulindac*

Diclofenac

Naproxen

Selective COX II inhibitors: *Celecoxib, rofecoxib*

Non-narcotic analgesics

NSAIDs are a group of chemically distinct compounds that act by inhibiting the enzyme COX. They are so named to distinguish them from the steroids, which also have anti-inflammatory actions. All NSAIDs have some degree of antipyretic, analgesic, and anti-inflammatory activity, but the relative proportion of each of these activities varies from drug to drug.

Aspirin

Indications and Usage

- Relief of fever and pain due to gout, rheumatic fever, rheumatoid arthritis, and common musculoskeletal trauma or irritation
- Prophylactic *inhibition of platelet aggregation* to decrease the incidence of cardiovascular ischemic attack
- Induction of *patent ductus arteriosus* closure in neonates. PGE_2 prevents closure of the ductus arteriosus; therefore, inhibition of its production results in closure of this patent shunt.
- Treatment for *dysmenorrhea*, which is caused (in part) by prostaglandin release from the endometrium

Mechanism of Action—Nonselective, irreversible inhibition of COX, resulting in decreased prostaglandin and thromboxane production. By blocking prostaglandin synthesis at thermoregulatory centers in the hypothalamus, *aspirin* (and all other NSAIDs) also acts as an antipyretic. (*See previous section for information about aspirin's antiplatelet actions.*)

Side Effects—**Gastric irritation and bleeding** are the most common and important. Prolonged bleeding time, respiratory depression, hyperthermia, and metabolic acidosis can also occur.

Propionic Acid Derivatives

Ibuprofen, fenoprofen, ketoprofen, oxaprozin

Indications and Usage—Relief of pain, especially due to rheumatoid arthritis and osteoarthritis

Mechanism of Action—**Reversible**, nonselective inhibitors of COX

Side Effects—Gastrointestinal irritation and bleeding, headache, **tinnitus, renal failure**

Indoleacetic Acids

Indomethacin, sulindac

Indications and Usage—Postoperative pain relief, fever refractory to other drugs, delay of labor by suppression of uterine contractions

Mechanism of Action—Reversible, nonselective inhibition of COX

Side Effects—GI ulcers, headache, dizziness, vertigo. Also hepatitis, acute pancreatitis, neutropenia, thrombocytopenia, and aplastic anemia

Diclofenac

Indications and Usage—Rheumatoid arthritis, osteoarthritis, ankylosing spondylitis

Mechanism of Action—Nonselective COX inhibitor

Side Effects—GI bleeding, elevation of hepatic enzymes

Naproxen

Indications and Usage—Inflammatory pains, menstrual cramping, osteoarthritis

Mechanism of Action—Nonselective COX inhibitor

Side Effects—GI bleeding

Selective COX II Inhibitors

Celecoxib, rofecoxib

Indications and Usage—Pain relief for osteoarthritis and rheumatoid arthritis

HARDCORE

Prostaglandins sensitize pain receptors to chemical and mechanical stimuli, and also act on the thermoregulatory center to cause fever.

HARDCORE

Aspirin should be avoided in children because of the risk of Reye's syndrome. If *aspirin* is given during a viral infection, children can develop fatal, fulminating hepatitis with cerebral edema.

HARDCORE

Propionic acid derivatives are widely used for chronic pain relief because their gastrointestinal side effects are less intense than those of aspirin.

HARDCORE

Indomethacin has a 100% hypersensitivity cross-reactivity with *aspirin*. The hypersensitivity consists of rashes, urticaria, and acute asthmatic attack.

HARDCORE

Concurrent administration of indomethacin may decrease the therapeutic effects of furosemide, thiazide diuretics, β-blockers, and ACE inhibitors.

HARDCORE

COX II inhibitors do not greatly inhibit platelet aggregation, since COX I is the predominant COX subtype present in platelets, and therefore COX II selective inhibitors do not have a large effect on bleeding time.

HARDCORE

The incidence of gastroduodenal ulcers in patients taking COX II inhibitors is <u>double</u> that of the regular population, but only <u>one-fourth</u> of those taking *ibuprofen* and *naproxen*.

HARDCORE

Acetaminophen is inactivated in peripheral tissues and has **no** local anti-inflammatory actions.

HARDCORE

N-*acetylcysteine* is used to treat *acetaminophen* overdose and acts by increasing glutathione levels in the liver and neutralizing free radicals produced by *acetaminophen* metabolites.

HARDCORE

Probenecid also blocks the tubular secretion of *penicillin* and is used to increase levels of the antibiotic.

HARDCORE

Allopurinol interferes with the metabolism of 6-*mercaptopurine* and *azathioprine*, therefore requires a lower dose of these medications.

HARDCORE

If given during acute gouty attack, *allopurinol* has the potential to actually **exacerbate** the condition.

Mechanism of Action—**Selective inhibition of the COX II enzyme**. As stated previously, COX has several isoforms, including COX I and COX II. Both subtypes are constitutively expressed in various tissues. However, COX II is also inducible and is up-regulated during inflammation and pain. Selective inhibition of COX II allows COX I to continue to produce prostaglandins not involved in the inflammatory response, especially in the stomach, where COX I products are responsible for mucous secretion. Thus, COX II inhibitors have fewer GI side effects than nonselective COX inhibitors.

Side Effects—Increased incidence of serious cardiovascular side effects (under investigation); abdominal pain, diarrhea, dyspepsia, renal toxicity.

Non-Narcotic Analgesics

 Acetaminophen

Indications and Usage—Fever, pain relief, dysmenorrhea

Mechanism of Action—Probably **inhibits (reversibly) prostaglandin synthesis in the CNS**

Side Effects—Excess *acetaminophen* depletes glutathione and forms toxic metabolites that can cause **hepatic necrosis**

DRUGS USED TO TREAT GOUT

Colchicine, probenecid, sulfinpyrazone, allopurinol

Gout is a chronic metabolic disease characterized by the deposit of urate crystals in joint spaces. As plasma and extracellular fluids become supersaturated with uric acid, urate crystals form and deposit within the joints and other soft tissues. Clinically this leads to the development of acute inflammatory arthritis, tenosynovitis, and the deposit of **tophi**, or aggregates of crystals surrounded by inflammation. Joints, tendons, and other connective tissues (e.g., antihelix of the ear) are common sites. The pharmacologic treatments for patients suffering from gout are directed at decreasing uric acid synthesis, increasing uric acid excretion, and decreasing the inflammatory reactions associated with this disorder. Be aware that NSAIDs are clinically the first line treatment for patients suffering from gout.

Colchicine

Indications and Usage—Acute attacks of gout

Mechanism of Action—Three major actions:

1. Blocks cell division by **binding mitotic spindles**
2. Binds tubulin decreasing the mobility of granulocytes into affected areas
3. Inhibits the synthesis and release of leukotrienes

Side Effects—Abdominal pain, **agranulocytosis**, **aplastic anemia**, alopecia

Probenecid and Sulfinpyrazone

Indications and Usage—Prophylaxis to prevent attacks of gout

Mechanism of Action—**Inhibits uric acid reabsorption** in the proximal tubule

Side Effects—Headache, anorexia, nausea

Allopurinol

Indications and Usage—Chronic suppression of gouty attacks, treatment of hyperuricemia secondary to renal disease or malignancies

Mechanism of Action—Competitively **inhibits xanthine oxidase**, the enzyme responsible for uric acid biosynthesis. The benefit of *allopurinol* is slow in onset.

Side Effects—Skin rash

HARDCORE REVIEW – HEMATOLOGICAL PHARMACOLOGY

TABLE 5-1 Antithrombus Therapeutics

Drug Class	Drugs	Mechanism of Action	Major Side Effects
Platelet function inhibitors	Aspirin	Irreversible COX I/II inhibitor	GI bleeding
	Abciximab	Binds and inhibits glycoprotein IIb/IIIa	Bleeding
	Dipyridamole	Phosphodiesterase inhibitor	Bleeding
	Ticlopidine, clopidogrel	Irreversibly inhibits ADP	Bleeding, neutropenia
Anticoagulants	Heparin	Binds ATIII, inhibiting thrombin (aPTT)	Bleeding, thrombocytopenia
	Enoxaparin, dalteparin	Binds ATIII, inhibiting thrombin	Bleeding
	Warfarin	Inhibits vitamin K epoxide reductase and factors II, VII, IX, and X (PT/INR)	Bleeding
Thrombolytics	Alteplase (tPA)	Converts plasminogen to plasmin	Bleeding
	Streptokinase	Converts plasminogen to plasmin	Bleeding, hypersensitivity
	Urokinase	Degrades both fibrin and fibrinogen	Bleeding

TABLE 5-2 Anti-Inflammatory Therapeutics (NSAIDs)

Drug Class	Drugs	Mechanism of Action	Major Side Effects
Aspirin		Irreversible COX I/II inhibitor	GI bleeding
Propionic acid derivatives	Ibuprofen, fenoprofen, ketoprofen, oxaprozin	Reversible, nonselective COX I/II inhibitor	GI bleeding, tinnitus, renal failure
Indoleacetic acids	Indomethacin, sulindac	Reversible, nonselective COX I/II inhibitor	GI ulcers, vertigo, hepatitis
Diclofenac		COX inhibitor	GI bleed, elevation of hepatic enzymes
Naproxen		COX inhibitor	GI bleeding
COX II inhibitors	Celecoxib, rofecoxib	Selective inhibition of COX II	GI bleeding
Non-narcotic analgesics	Acetaminophen	COX inhibitor in CNS	Hepatic toxicity

TABLE 5-3 Antigout Therapeutics

Drugs	Mechanism of Action	Major Side Effects
Colchicine	Binds mitotic spindles and tubulin and inhibits release of leukotrienes	Agranulocytosis, aplastic anemia, alopecia
Probenecid, sulfinpyrazone	Inhibits renal uric acid reabsorption in proximal tubule	Headache, anorexia
Allopurinol	Inhibits uric acid synthesis	Skin rash

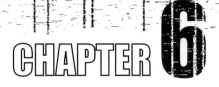

Pulmonary Pharmacology

Pulmonary pharmacology on the USMLE Step 1 exam focuses primarily on the symptomatic treatment of asthma. You should also be familiar with the pharmacological management of rhinitis and cough.

ASTHMA AND OBSTRUCTIVE LUNG DISORDERS

Chronic obstructive pulmonary disorder (COPD) is a persistent lung disorder characterized by reduced maximal expiratory flow and slow forced emptying of the lungs that is only minimally reversible with bronchodilators. Asthma is typically not considered a form of COPD, because asthmatic symptoms can be reversed. Asthma is a pulmonary airway disorder characterized by hyperresponsiveness of the bronchioles, inflammation, and bronchoconstriction. In the asthmatic patient, the large conducting airways narrow abnormally and become chronically inflamed in response to allergens, infections, psychological stressors, or for unknown reasons. These irritants induce an inflammatory response involving the infiltration of eosinophils and release of cytotoxic mediators that damage the ciliated respiratory epithelial cells. This airway irritation and inflammation cause bronchospasm and the clinical characteristics of asthma: *cough, dyspnea, and wheezing.*

Bronchiolar diameter is controlled by several opposing systems. Stimulation of bronchial β_2-receptors produces an increase in intracellular cAMP levels and results in bronchodilation (Figure 6-1). Simulation of bronchial muscarinic receptors results in a decrease in intracellular cAMP levels, and causes bronchoconstriction and increased secretions (Figure 6-1). Although current asthma treatments are not curative, they can diminish asthmatic symptoms by:

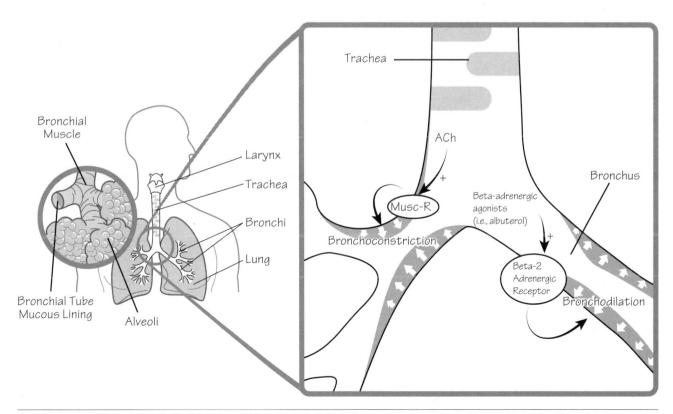

Figure 6-1 Overview of the mechanisms leading to bronchoconstriction and bronchodilation in the lungs. Acetylcholine (ACh) stimulates muscarinic receptors (M) located on airway smooth muscle, resulting in bronchoconstriction. Stimulation of β_2-adrenergic receptors (β_2-AR) results in relaxation of airway smooth muscle and bronchodilation.

1. **Promoting bronchodilation** (β₂-adrenergic receptor agonists)
2. **Suppression of the inflammatory response and muscarinic receptor mediated bronchoconstriction** (anti-inflammatory agents and anticholinergics)

β-Adrenergic Receptor Agonists

Nonselective β-adrenergic receptor agonists: *Isoproterenol, epinephrine*
Inhaled β₂-adrenergic receptor selective agonists: *Albuterol, terbutaline, salmeterol*

Nonselective β-Adrenergic Receptor Agonists

Isoproterenol, epinephrine

Indications and Usage—Acute asthma attacks

Mechanism of Action—Agonist at both β₁- and β₂-adrenergic receptors. β₂-adrenergic receptor activation results in bronchial smooth muscle relaxation and *bronchodilation*.

Side Effects—β₁-adrenergic receptor activation can result in tachycardia, anxiety, fear, headache, and tremor.

Inhaled β₂-Selective Agonists

SHORT-ACTING AND FAST ONSET

Albuterol, terbutaline

Indications and Usage—Acute asthma attacks and prevention of exercise-induced asthma

Mechanism of Action—β₂-adrenergic receptor activation results in bronchial smooth muscle relaxation and *bronchodilation*.

Side Effects—Tremors and tachycardia due to activation of β₁-adrenergic receptors; *hypokalemia* can occur at high doses due to a β₂-adrenergic receptor-mediated increase in the cellular uptake of serum potassium

LONG-ACTING AND SLOW ONSET

Salmeterol

Indications and Usage—Prophylactic treatment of moderate persistent asthma, particularly useful for patients with *nocturnal symptoms*

Mechanism of Action—β₂-adrenergic receptor activation results in bronchial smooth muscle relaxation and *bronchodilation*.

Side Effects—β₁-adrenergic receptor activation can cause tremors and tachycardia; hypokalemia can occur at high doses.

Receptor Antagonists and Enzyme Inhibitors

Methylxanthines: *Theophylline, caffeine*
Muscarinic antagonists: *Ipratropium, oxitropium*
Antileukotrienes: *Zileuton, montelukast, zafirlukast*
Mast-cell stabilizers: *Cromolyn*
Corticosteroids: *Prednisone, prednisolone, beclomethasone, fluticasone*

Methylxanthines

Theophylline, caffeine

Indications and Usage—Chronic and nocturnal asthma

Mechanism of Action—Methylxanthines act by *inhibiting the enzyme phosphodiesterase (PDE)*. PDE (type IV) is responsible for degrading intracellular cAMP, resulting in an increase in intracellular cAMP levels in smooth muscle and *bronchodilation*.

Side Effects—Arrhythmias, seizures, GI irritation, and various *drug interactions*

Muscarinic Antagonists

Ipratropium, oxitropium

Indications and Usage—In asthmatics unable to tolerate adrenergic agonists, or in combination with β₂ agonists for *chronic bronchitis and COPD*

HARDCORE

Anaphylaxis is a generalized allergic reaction that is associated with systemic distribution of an allergen. Treatment of anaphylaxis involves injection of epinephrine, followed by use of antihistamines and steroids.

HARDCORE

Albuterol is the *drug of choice for acute asthma attacks*.

HARDCORE

Remember that *albuterol* and *terbutaline* are *selective* for β₂-adrenergic receptors, meaning that they preferentially bind β₂-adrenergic receptors over other β-adrenergic receptor subtypes. However, they still have some activity at β₁-adrenergic receptors, albeit less than nonselective β-adrenergic receptor agonists, which can result in tachycardia and tremors.

HARDCORE

Methylxanthines also have anti-inflammatory actions.

HARDCORE

Theophylline has a very *narrow therapeutic window* and may cause nausea, insomnia, cardiac arrhythmias, and convulsions.

Mechanism of Action—Blockade of parasympathetic-mediated bronchoconstriction via nonselective muscarinic receptor antagonism

Side Effects—Rare, but may include typical anticholinergic side effects, including dry mouth, vision changes, tachycardia, and urinary retention

Antileukotrienes

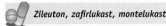 *Zileuton, zafirlukast, montelukast*

Leukotrienes increase vascular permeability and promote chemotaxis of inflammatory mediators, resulting in **increased mucous production, edema, and bronchoconstriction**.

ZILEUTON

Indications and Usage—Long-term asthma prophylaxis

Mechanism of Action—**Inhibition of 5-lipooxygenase**, resulting in decreased formation of leukotrienes

Side Effects—Hepatotoxicity, headaches, indigestion

ZAFIRLUKAST AND MONTELUKAST

Indications and Usage—Long-term asthma prophylaxis

Mechanism of Action—**Inhibition of the leukotriene D4 and E4 receptors**

Side Effects—Hepatotoxicity, pharyngitis, headache

Mast Cell Stabilizer

 Cromolyn sodium

Indications and Usage—Prophylaxis and prevention of inflammation in asthmatic patients

Mechanism of Action—Mast cells secrete histamine and play a role in defending against parasitic and bacterial infections and in immediate hypersensitivity responses, such as asthma, rhinitis, urticaria, and anaphylaxis. Mast cell stabilizers **prevent mast cell degranulation**, thereby inhibiting the release of histamine and other inflammatory mediators. *Cromolyn* also subdues alveolar macrophages and suppresses the response of exposed irritant nerves.

Side Effects—Cough, wheezing, larynx irritation

Corticosteroids

 Prednisone, prednisolone, beclomethasone, fluticasone

Indications and Usage—Mild, moderate, or severe asthma that is resistant to other treatments

Mechanism of Action—**Inhibits the enzyme phospholipase-A₂**, resulting in a decrease in the production of prostaglandins and leukotrienes and suppression of the chronic inflammatory response of asthma

Side Effects—**Exogenous Cushing's syndrome**: fluid retention, fat redistribution (buffalo hump and moon facies), predisposition for infections, poor wound healing, glucose intolerance, and adrenal insufficiency

RHINITIS

Rhinitis is inflammation of the mucous membrane of the nose. Patients with rhinitis experience nasal congestion, watery rhinorrhea, and sneezing. The treatment of rhinitis involves blocking the action of mediators released by mast cells, including histamine, leukotrienes, and chemotactic agents.

Antihistamines

SEDATING ANTIHISTAMINES

 Diphenhydramine, chlorpheniramine, hydroxyzine, cetirizine

Mechanism of Action—H₁-histamine receptor blocker that targets the symptoms of histamine release (bronchiolar spasm, mucosal thickening, and cellular infiltration)

Side Effects—Sedation

NONSEDATING ANTIHISTAMINES

 Loratadine, desloratadine, fexofenadine

Mechanism of Action—H₁-histamine receptor blocker that targets the symptoms of histamine release

HARDCORE

Ipratropium and oxitropium are charged analogs of *atropine*, and do not cross the blood-brain barrier.

HARDCORE

Antileukotrienes are not used for the reversal of an acute asthma attack.

HARDCORE

Antilukotrines are often used with corticosteroids to improve asthma control and reduce corticosteroid dosage.

HARDCORE

Mast cell stabilizers are less effective than *corticosteroids* for long-term prophylaxis.

HARDCORE

To be effective, cromolyn sodium should be administered shortly before exposure to a possible asthma precipitating factor.

HARDCORE

Cromolyn sodium is not for use in the reversal of an acute asthma attack.

HARDCORE

Oral corticosteroids are reserved for severe asthmatics that are unresponsive to other therapies. These agents are sparingly used because of the wide spectrum of systemic side effects associated with chronic use.

HARDCORE

Side effects of aerosol steroid use include hoarse voice and *Candida* overgrowth in the mouth (thrush).

HARDCORE

Corticosteroid therapy can result in impairment of the hypothalamic-pituitary-adrenal axis, and a decrease in the size of the adrenal cortex (adrenal insufficiency).

HARDCORE

Sedation is not associated with non-sedating antihistamines, because they do not readily enter the CNS.

HARDCORE

Corticosteroids can be administered as aerosols, which decrease systemic side effects, but result in a shorter duration of action.

HARDCORE

Treatment of chronic rhinitis with corticosteroids may not show improvement for up to 2 weeks after starting therapy.

HARDCORE

Dextromethorphan does not penetrate the blood-brain barrier as readily as other opioids and is, therefore, not as great of an addiction liability as other opioids.

HARDCORE

To treat cough, these drugs do not require doses high enough to produce analgesia.

Side Effects—Slightly increased risk of viral infection

α-Adrenergic Receptor Agonists

> *Phenylephrine, pseudoephedrine, oxymetazoline*

Mechanism of Action—Stimulate α_1-adrenergic receptors, resulting in the constriction of dilated arterioles, thereby reducing arteriole leakage and congestion

Side Effects—Increased blood pressure, rebound nasal congestion (if used for extended periods)

Corticosteroids

> *Prednisone, prednisolone, beclomethasone, fluticasone*

Indications and Usage—Rhinitis

Mechanism of Action—***Inhibits the enzyme phospholipase-A_2***, resulting in a decrease in the production of prostaglandins and leukotrienes and suppression of inflammation

COUGH

Cough is a complex interaction between peripheral stimuli and cough centers in the CNS. Each cough occurs through the stimulation of a complex reflex arc. The cough reflex can be initiated by irritation of cough receptors in the upper or lower respiratory tracts, the pericardium, esophagus, diaphragm, or stomach, or through mechanical cough receptors stimulated by touch or displacement. Impulses from cough receptors travel to the "cough center" in the brainstem. The cough center generates an efferent signal that travels to expiratory musculature, producing the cough. Drugs used to treat cough (antitussives) act by decreasing the sensitivity of peripheral sensory receptors or by inhibiting the basic cough circuitry in the brainstem.

Opioid Antagonists

> *Codeine, dextromethorphan*

Mechanism of Action—The exact mechanism of opioid antitussives is unknown, but it likely involves both peripheral and central actions.

Side Effects—Respiratory and CNS depression, euphoria, constipation

HARDCORE REVIEW – PULMONARY PHARMACOLOGY

Some *hardcore* points you should remember about asthma:

- Short-acting β_2 agonists (e.g., *albuterol*) are first line for an acute asthma exacerbation
- Steroids (*prednisone*), mast cell stabilizers (*cromolyn*), methylxanthines (*theophylline*), antileukotrienes (*zileuton, montelukast, zafirlukast*), and long-acting β_2 agonists (*salmeterol*) are effective for prophylactic and long-term treatment of asthma. They are not useful in treatment of acute asthma attacks, because their effects are not immediate.
- Nonselective β-blockers (*propranolol*) are contraindicated in patients with COPD (including asthma), because they can cause bronchoconstriction.
- Most agents used in the treatment of asthma are inhaled, since this method delivers the drug directly to the lung, resulting in fewer systemic side effects and a more rapid onset of action.
- β_2-adrenergic receptor stimulation leads to an increase in cAMP, causing bronchodilation
- Muscarinic acetylcholine receptor stimulation leads to a decrease in cAMP, causing bronchoconstriction.

TABLE 6-1	Drugs Used to Treat Asthma

DRUG CLASS	DRUGS	MECHANISM OF ACTION	MAJOR SIDE EFFECTS
β₂ agonists			
Nonselective β agonists	*Isoproterenol, epinephrine*	β_1/β_2-Receptor agonist	Tachycardia
Inhaled β₂-selective agonists: Short-acting and fast onset	*Albuterol, terbutaline*	β_2-Receptor agonist	Tachycardia
Inhaled β₂-selective agonists: Long-acting and slow onset	*Salmeterol*	β_2-Receptor agonist	Tachycardia
Methylxanthines	*Theophylline*	PDE inhibitor, increases cAMP levels	Drug interactions, arrhythmias
Muscarinic antagonists	*Ipratropium, oxitropium*	Muscarinic receptor antagonists	Dry mouth, urinary retention
Antileukotrienes	*Zileuton*	5-lipooxygenase inhibitor	Hepatotoxicity
	Zafirlukast, montelukast	Cysteinyl-leukotriene 1 receptor inhibitor	Hepatotoxicity
Cromolyn	*Cromolyn*	Mast cell stabilizer	Larynx irritation
Corticosteroids	*Prednisone, prednisolone, beclomethasone, fluticasone*	Phospholipase-A₂ enzyme inhibitor	Cushing's (systemic); *Candida* (inhaled)

TABLE 6-2	Drugs Used to Treat Rhinitis

DRUG CLASS	DRUGS	MECHANISM OF ACTION	MAJOR SIDE EFFECTS
Antihistamines			
Sedating antihistamines	*Diphenhydramine, chlorpheniramine, hydroxyzine, cetirizine*	H₁-histamine receptor blocker	Sedation
Nonating antihistamines	*Loratadine, desloratadine, fexofenadine*	H₁-histamine receptor blocker (less CNS entry)	
α agonists	*Phenylephrine, pseudoephedrine, oxymetazoline*	α_1-Receptor agonist	Increased blood pressure, rebound nasal congestion

TABLE 6-3	Drugs Acting on CNS Cough Centers

DRUG CLASS	DRUG NAMES	MECHANISM OF ACTION	MAJOR SIDE EFFECTS
Opiate/opioid derivatives	*Codeine, hydrocodone, hydromorphone, dextromethorphan*	Suppress cough center	CNS/respiratory depression (except *dextromethorphan*)

CHAPTER 7

Endocrine Pharmacology

The focus of Step 1 endocrine pharmacology typically centers on the oral treatment of diabetes. Also included in this chapter are sex hormones, corticosteroids, drugs used to treat osteoporosis, hormones of the pituitary gland, and thyroid hormones.

DIABETES MELLITUS

Diabetes mellitus is characterized by a group of disorders resulting from deficient insulin secretory responses, glucose underutilization, and hyperglycemia. This disorder can be divided into two primary classifications, **type I and type II**, based on etiology, age of onset, and insulin dependence.

- **Type I diabetes** is characterized by an absolute lack of insulin caused by the loss of pancreatic insulin-producing beta cells. This disease occurs early in life, commonly following an autoimmune-mediated loss of pancreatic beta cells. These patients do not produce endogenous insulin, and injectable insulin therapy is the only effective treatment. Type I diabetes is also referred to as **insulin-dependent diabetes mellitus (IDDM)**. Without proper insulin therapy, **diabetic ketoacidosis (DKA)** may develop, creating a clinical picture that includes nausea, vomiting, electrolyte imbalance, Kussmaul breathing (deep, rapid respiration characteristic of diabetic or other causes of acidosis), coma, and possibly death.

- **Type II diabetes**, the more common variety of diabetes, is also called **noninsulin-dependent diabetes mellitus (NIDDM)**. Generally, this disease arises later in life as a result of insulin resistance at peripheral tissues. Although people with this condition suffer from abnormally elevated levels of blood glucose, they typically are still able to produce insulin. This allows for more therapeutic options, including medications that decrease the absorption of glucose from the intestinal tract, reduce serum glucagon levels, increase the sensitivity of peripheral tissues to insulin, and stimulate increased insulin release from the pancreas.

Without adequate long-term treatment of both types of diabetes, patients can develop serious problems, including microvascular complications (cardiomyopathy, retinopathy, and nephropathy) and macrovascular complications (atherosclerosis, peripheral vascular disease, stroke, and renal failure).

DRUGS USED TO TREAT DIABETES MELLITUS

The Step 1 exam focuses primarily on the mechanism and side effects of the oral hypoglycemic agents; however, you should also be familiar with the different types of insulin preparations.

Insulin

A variety of insulin preparations have been developed to provide insulin dependent diabetics with a means of insulin replacement (see Figure 7-1). These patients are able to achieve glucose control with multiple daily injections of insulin preparations. These preparations differ in their duration of action and other pharmacokinetic characteristics. Be aware that the *most important side effect of insulin is hypoglycemia*, which may lead to coma and seizures. Short-acting preparations are typically injected shortly before meals to mimic the physiologic bolus of insulin typically seen in normal individuals after meals. Intermediate- and long-acting preparations are typically injected at bedtime to mimic the basal insulin output seen in normal individuals.

Indications and Usage—Type I (insulin-dependent) diabetes; type II diabetes patients who have advanced disease or are refractory to oral hypoglycemic agents

Mechanism of Action—Insulin preparations produce the same physiological actions as endogenous insulin, primarily the reduction of blood glucose.

There are many different insulin preparations available:

Rapid/Short-Acting Preparations

These act within minutes and are composed of recombinant human insulin.

HARDCORE

When endogenous or prepared insulin binds to an insulin receptor, it induces the phosphorylation of tyrosine kinase and the activation of intracellular signaling cascades (DAG, IP3, and PIP2 are all involved). These signals result in the translocation of glucose transporters from endosomal compartments to the plasma membrane and an increase in glucose uptake.

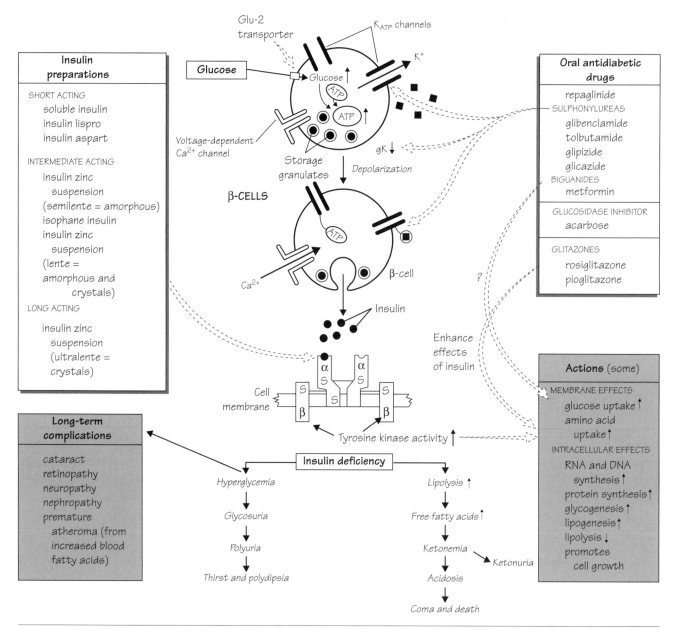

Figure 7-1 Overview of the antidiabetic agents. (Reprinted with permission from Neal MJ. Medical Pharmacology at a Glance. 4th ed. Oxford: Blackwell Publishing, 2002:78.)

HARDCORE

Remember: "Regular" is *Rapid*

HARDCORE

Regular insulin is the only insulin preparation that can be administered intravenously.

HARDCORE

Lispro insulin is commonly used in conjunction with a longer-acting insulin to achieve appropriate glucose control.

HARDCORE

"*Lente*" means "*slow*" in Latin.

Regular Insulin
This insulin is a soluble, crystalline zinc insulin.

Lispro Insulin
This insulin preparation is the ***most rapidly absorbed*** insulin after subcutaneous injection.

Intermediate-Acting Preparations
These have a more gradual onset than short acting insulin preparations.

Semilente
The onset of action and peak response of this insulin are fairly rapid, but slower than regular insulin.

Isophane or NPH
Less soluble than other preparations, these result in an intermediate onset and duration of action.

Lente
This preparation is a combination of *semilente* (30%) and *ultralente* (70%; see below). This combination allows for relatively fast onset and a prolonged duration of action.

Long-Acting Preparations
These preparations have a slower onset of action and a longer duration of action.

TABLE 7-1	Insulin Preparations		
INSULIN PREPARATION	**ONSET (HR)**	**PEAK (HR)**	**DURATION (HR)**
Rapid-acting			
Insulin lispro	Within 15 min	$1/2$–$1^1/2$	3–5
Insulin aspart	Within 10 min	1–3	3–5
Short-acting			
Regular	$1/2$–1	2–4	5–8
Intermediate-acting			
NPH	1–2	6–14	12+
Lente	1–3	6–14	12+
Long-acting			
Ultralente	6	18–24	24+
Insulin glargine	$1^1/2$	Flat	24

(Reprinted with permission from Yang KY. Blueprints Notes & Cases: Pharmacology. Malden, MA: Blackwell Publishing, 2004:62.)

ULTRALENTE

This preparation is composed of large particles that absorb slowly, producing a slower-onset, longer-lasting response.

INSULIN GLARGINE

This is one of the most commonly used preparations due to its rapid onset of action, relatively constant rate of release (i.e., no peaks or troughs), and **long duration of action**.

Oral Hypoglycemic Agents

> **Sulfonylureas:** *Tolbutamide, glyburide, glipizide, chlorpropamide*
> **Biguanide:** *Metformin*
> **Glitazones:** *Rosiglitazone, pioglitazone*
> **α-Glucosidase inhibitor:** *Acarbose*

Most patients with type II diabetes mellitus respond well to oral hypoglycemic agents and, therefore, do not need to use the various insulin preparations described previously. These agents are only for type II patients who have some capacity to produce endogenous insulin. These agents work by a variety of mechanisms to achieve the same goal: **to lower blood glucose to a normal (or acceptable) level**.

Sulfonylureas

> **First generation:** *Tolbutamide, chlorpropamide*
> **Second generation:** *Glyburide, glipizide*

Mechanism of Action—Both first and second-generation *sulfonylureas* work in three ways:

1. **Improve the binding of circulating insulin** to target tissues and receptors
2. **Stimulate insulin release** from pancreatic beta cells by inhibiting K^+ channels. This causes the depolarization and subsequent activation of voltage-sensitive Ca^{2+} channels, leading to an increased insulin release.
3. **Reduce serum glucagon levels**

Side Effects—**Hypoglycemia**, hyponatremia, hypokalemia

Biguanide

> *Metformin*

Mechanism of Action

- Increases glucose uptake into cells
- **Inhibits gluconeogenesis**, resulting in a decrease in hepatic glucose output

Side Effects—**Lactic acidosis** (anion-gap metabolic acidosis)

Glitazones

> *Rosiglitazone, pioglitazone*

HARDCORE

Sulfonylureas cause allergic reaction in patients with sulfa allergies: **SULF**onylurea = **SULF**a allergy.

HARDCORE

Sulfonylureas are **contraindicated in pregnant women**, because they can cross the placenta and deplete insulin from the fetal pancreas.

HARDCORE

Consumption of alcohol while taking *chlorpropamide* can induce a *disulfuram*-like reaction (severe nausea/vomiting) and hypotension.

HARDCORE

Sulfonylureas are contraindicated in patients with renal or hepatic insufficiency, because their accumulation may lead to a hypoglycemic episode.

HARDCORE

Metformin decreases circulating levels of LDL and VLDL and increases HDL levels.

HARDCORE

Patients on *metformin* will often **lose weight**, so it is considered the *hardcore* drug of choice in newly diagnosed type II diabetics.

HARDCORE

Metformin does **not produce allergic reactions** in patients allergic to sulfa drugs.

Mechanism of Action—Increases the sensitivity of peripheral tissue to circulating insulin

Side Effects—Weight gain, hepatotoxicity

α-Glucosidase Inhibitors

Acarbose, miglitol

Mechanism of Action—***Inhibits the enzyme α-glucosidase***, which hydrolyzes polysaccharides in the intestinal brush border. Inhibition of this enzyme leads to decreased absorption of starches and polysaccharides, and a decreased plasma glucose level following a meal.

Side Effects—Flatulence, diarrhea, abdominal cramping

STEROID HORMONES

Estrogens: *Estradiol, estriol, estrone, ethinyl estradiol, diethylstilbestrol (DES)*
Antiestrogens: *Clomiphene, tamoxifen, raloxifene*
Progestins: *Medroxyprogesterone, hydroxyprogesterone, norethindrone, norgestrel*
Antiprogestins: *Mifepristone*
Androgens: *Testosterone, danazol, nandrolone, stanozolol, fluoxymesterone*
Antiandrogens: *Finasteride, flutamide, ketoconazole/spironolactone*

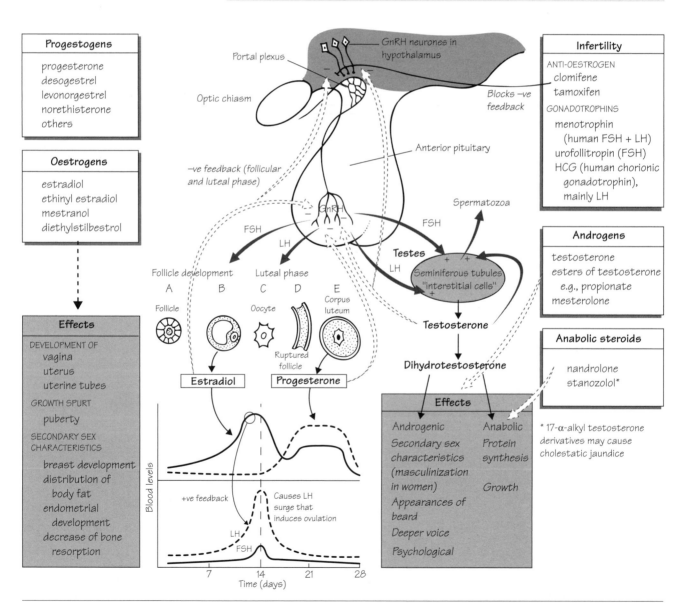

Figure 7-2 **Overview of sex hormones and therapeutics.** (Reprinted with permission from Neal MJ. Medical Pharmacology at a Glance. 4th ed. Oxford: Blackwell Publishing, 2002:74.)

Sex hormones are produced endogenously by the gonads and adrenals and are important for conception, embryonic maturation, and the development of secondary sexual characteristics at puberty. Pharmacologically, sex hormones and sex hormone antagonists are used for a wide variety of medical conditions. Focus on the key differences in target tissues, therapeutic actions, and side effect profiles of each hormone/drug class. Specific combinations of agents (e.g., combination oral contraceptives) are outside the scope of the board examination.

Estrogens

 Estradiol, estriol, estrone, ethinyl estradiol, DES

Indications and Usage—Contraception, postmenopausal hormone therapy, hypogonadism

Mechanism of Action—Bind estrogen receptors, resulting in the activation of hormone-specific RNA synthesis, and, ultimately, a physiologic response

Side Effects—Nausea, vomiting, ***venous thromboembolism (clotting)***, breast tenderness

Antiestrogens

 Clomiphene, tamoxifen, raloxifene

CLOMIPHENE

Indications and Usage—Stimulation of ovulation in cases of infertility associated with anovulation

Mechanism of Action—At low doses, *clomiphene* acts as a competitive antagonist/partial agonist at estrogen receptors, blocking the negative feedback of estrogens on the hypothalamus and pituitary. This results in an ***increased secretion of gonadotropin-releasing hormone (GnRH)*** and the stimulation of ovulation.

Side Effects—Ovarian enlargement, vasomotor flushes, visual disturbances, ***multiple pregnancies*** (fertilization of multiple ova)

TAMOXIFEN AND RALOXIFENE

Indications and Usage—Estrogen receptor-positive breast cancer, osteoporosis (primarily *raloxifene*)

Mechanism of Action—These drugs are competitive antagonists at estrogen receptors.

Side Effects—Induces a low estrogen state, therefore side effects mimic menopause including: hot flashes, nausea, vomiting, and vaginal bleeding

Progestins

 Medroxyprogesterone, hydroxyprogesterone, norethindrone, norgestrel

Indications and Usage—Contraception, endometriosis, dysmenorrhea, dysfunctional uterine bleeding, endometrial carcinoma

Mechanism of Action—Binds progestin receptors, resulting in the activation of hormone-specific RNA synthesis, and, ultimately, a physiologic response

Side Effects—Edema, depression, weight gain

Antiprogestins

 Mifepristone (RU-486)

Indications and Usage—***Abortion of fetus in very early pregnancy***, contraception

Mechanism of Action—Antagonizes the effect of progesterone at progestin receptors, preventing implantation of the embryo, and resulting in abortion of the fetus

Side Effects—Uterine bleeding

Androgens

 Testosterone, danazol, nandrolone, stanozolol, fluoxymesterone

Indications and Usage—Hypogonadism; anabolic effects for burn victims; senile osteoporosis; growth in boys with pituitary dwarfism; endometriosis

Mechanism of Action—Binds testosterone receptors, resulting in the activation of hormone-specific RNA synthesis, and, ultimately, a physiologic response

Side Effects

- Cholestatic jaundice, liver abnormalities, hepatocellular carcinoma
- Masculinization in females
- Can be converted in vivo to estrogen, resulting in priapism, impotence, gynecomastia, decreased spermatogenesis in males
- Abnormal sexual maturation and premature closing of epiphyseal plates in children (stunting of growth)

HARDCORE

In the past, postmenopausal hormone replacement therapy was thought to decrease the risk of atherosclerotic disease (by increasing HDL levels), prevent osteoporosis (due to decreases in osteoclast activity), diminish hot flashes, and alleviate atrophic vaginitis. However, recent studies indicate that the combination of estrogens/progestins taken longer than 5 years, in fact, increases the risk of heart attack, stroke, clotting (deep vein thrombosis and pulmonary emboli), and breast cancer.

HARDCORE

Synthetic agents (e.g., *ethinyl estradiol*) are used because they undergo less first-pass metabolism when taken orally (for both *estrogens* and *progestins*).

HARDCORE

DES has been linked to ***clear cell vaginal adenocarcinomas*** in daughters of women who took the drug during their pregnancy.

HARDCORE

Tamoxifen is an antagonist in breast tissue, but acts as a partial agonist and can stimulate estrogen receptors in endometrial, skeletal, and cardiovascular tissue. *Raloxifene* acts as an antagonist in both breast and endometrial tissue.

HARDCORE

Progestins increase LDL levels and decrease HDL levels.

HARDCORE

Progestins have also been associated with thrombophlebitis and pulmonary embolism.

HARDCORE

Outside of muscle and liver, testosterone (and testosterone analogs) must be converted to ***dihydrotestosterone (DHT) by 5-α-reductase to be active***.

HARDCORE

Androgens increase LDL levels and decrease HDL levels.

HARDCORE

Oral androgens may cause hepatotoxicity.

Antiandrogen

 Finasteride, flutamide, ketoconazole, leuprolide

FINASTERIDE

Indications and Usage—Benign prostatic hypertrophy (periurethral and transitional), baldness

Mechanism of Action—***Inhibits 5-α-reductase***, decreasing the formation of DHT by the prostate. This results in a reduction in the size of the prostate and a decrease in DHT-dependent hair loss.

Side Effects—Feminization

FLUTAMIDE

Indications and Usage—Prostate cancer (posterior and peripheral)

Mechanism of Action—***Competitively antagonizes the actions of androgens at target cells***, thereby decreasing tumor growth in testosterone-dependent prostate cancer.

Side Effects—Feminization

KETOCONAZOLE

Indications and Usage—Polycystic ovarian syndrome, antifungal

Mechanism of Action—Inhibition of cytochrome P450 enzymes involved in steroid synthesis

Side Effects—Pruritus, gynecomastia, hair loss, hemolytic anemia

LEUPROLIDE

Indications and Usage—Prostate cancer; endometriosis

Mechanism of Action—Leuprolide is a ***gonadotropin-releasing hormone (GnRH) agonist*** that inhibits the production of luteinizing hormone (LH) and follicle-stimulating hormone (FSH) by stimulating negative feedback at the hypothalamus. Inhibition of negative feedback results in a decrease in testosterone and estrogen levels.

Side Effects—Gynecomastia, weight gain, depression, hot flashes (women)

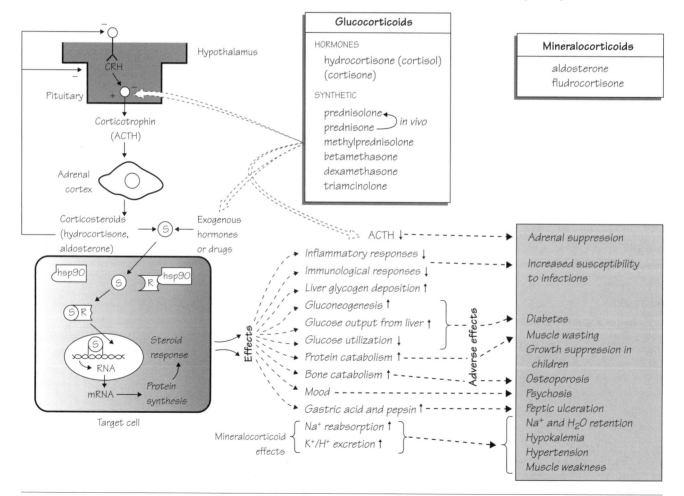

Figure 7-3 Corticosteroids. (Reprinted with permission from Neal MJ. Medical Pharmacology at a Glance. 4th ed. Oxford: Blackwell Publishing, 2002:72.)

CORTICOSTEROIDS

Short-acting glucocorticoids: *Hydrocortisone, cortisone*
Intermediate-acting glucocorticoids: *Prednisone, prednisolone, methylprednisone*
Long-acting glucocorticoids: *Betamethasone, dexamethasone*
Mineralocorticoids: *Fludrocortisone, deoxycorticosterone*

Indications and Usage—Inflammation, allergies, asthma, replacement therapy for adrenocortical insufficiency and congenital adrenal hyperplasia

Mechanism of Action—Bind to **intracellular cytoplasmic receptors**, resulting in **changes in gene transcription, and ultimately resulting in a physiologic response**. Since corticosteroids act by altering gene transcription, the time to effect is longer than with other drugs. Physiologic effects of corticosteroid administration include:

- Decreased plasma levels of eosinophils, basophils, monocytes, and lymphocytes
- Increased plasma levels of hemoglobin, erythrocytes, and platelets
- Increased plasma glucose levels
- Stimulation of protein catabolism and lipolysis
- Inhibition of phospholipase A_2, resulting in a decrease in leukotriene and prostaglandin production

Side Effects—**Cushing-like syndrome** (redistribution of body fat/truncal obesity, buffalo hump, moon facies, acne, insomnia), negative calcium balance, edema, hypertension, peptic ulcers, weight gain, easy bruising, myopathy

HARDCORE

Patients taking corticosteroids are at an increased risk of infection and impaired wound healing.

HARDCORE

When used chronically, patients can become dependent on corticosteroids. Abrupt cessation can result in psychosis and an acute adrenal insufficiency syndrome that can be fatal (due to hypotension and shock).

DRUGS USED TO TREAT OSTEOPOROSIS

Bisphosphonates: *Alendronate, pamidronate, risedronate*
Calcium carbonate
Calcitonin
Hormone replacement therapy: *Estrogen*

Osteoporosis is a condition of diminished bone matrix that occurs when the rate of bone formation (a function of *osteoblasts*) to bone resorption (a function of *osteoclasts*) is out of balance. This occurs with age, but may be accelerated by a premature loss of ovarian function, medications (*glucocorticosteroids*), or low dietary calcium intake. Drugs used to treat osteoporosis act to restore the balance between bone formation and resorption.

Bisphosphonates

Alendronate, pamidronate, risedronate

Mechanism of Action—Inhibit osteoclast activity and bone resorption

Side Effects—**Erosive esophageal damage**

Calcium Carbonate

Mechanism of Action—Supplementation of dietary calcium for use in bone formation

Side Effects—GI discomfort

Calcitonin

Mechanism of Action—Directly inhibits osteoclasts and bone resorption

Side Effects—Flushing, nausea, vomiting

Hormone Replacement Therapy: Estrogen

Mechanism of Action—Estrogen replacement therapy at the time of menopause inhibits osteoclast-mediated bone resorption, slowing bone loss and increasing bone density

Side Effects—Endometrial cancer if used without progestin replacement; increased risk of endometrial and breast cancer

HARDCORE

Patients should take vitamin D with calcium to facilitate intestinal calcium absorption.

HARDCORE

Pituitary hormones are not effective when administered orally, so they are delivered intranasally or injected.

PITUITARY HORMONES

Somatostatin, octreotide, leuprolide, oxytocin, vasopressin, desmopressin

Somatostatin and Octreotide

These drugs are synthetic somatostatin analogs.

Indications and Usage

- **Acromegaly** from hormone-secreting tumors
- **Dumping syndrome**: Occurs after eating in patients with shunts of the upper GI tract. It is characterized by flushing, sweating, dizziness, weakness, and vasomotor collapse. Dumping syndrome results from the rapid passage of large amounts of food into the small intestine, with an osmotic effect that removes fluid from the plasma and results in hypovolemia, pancreatitis, and gastrointestinal bleeding.

Mechanism of Action—Somatostatin is a naturally occurring hormone (and octreotide a synthetic analog) that inhibits the secretion of pituitary and gastrointestinal hormones including serotonin, gastrin, vasoactive intestinal peptide (VIP), insulin, glucagon, secretin, motilin, pancreatic polypeptide, growth hormone, and thyrotropin.

Side Effects—Flatulence, nausea, steatorrhea

Leuprolide

Indications and Usage—Infertility, prostate cancer, endometriosis, uterine fibroids

Mechanism of Action—An analog of GnRH that acts as a **GnRH antagonist**; at low doses *leuprolide* can act as a partial agonist

Side Effects—Nausea, vomiting

Oxytocin

Indications and Usage—***Stimulates uterine contraction to induce labor*** (given intravenously); promotes breast milk ejection (given intranasally)

Mechanism of Action—Contraction of uterine smooth muscle and of myoepithelial cells around mammary alveoli

Side Effects—Uncommon, but include hypertensive crisis, uterine rupture, and water retention

Vasopressin (Antidiuretic Hormone, ADH) and Desmopressin

Indications and Usage—Diabetes insipidus, nocturnal enuresis

Mechanism of Action—Binds to the V-2 receptor in the kidneys' collecting tubules, ***increasing water resorption***. V-1 receptors are linked to diacylglycerol-inositol 1,4,5-trisphosphate (DAG-IP$_3$), and their activation results in increasing intracellular cAMP levels. This also results in vasoconstriction.

Side Effects—Water intoxication and hyponatremia

THYROID HORMONES

Treatment of hypothyroidism: *Liothyronine, levothyroxine*

Treatment of hyperthyroidism: *Radioactive iodine, propylthiouracil, methimazole, iodide*

The thyroid gland maintains normal levels of metabolism in a variety of body tissues. For treatment, it is important to recognize the signs of **hypothyroidism** (bradycardia, cold intolerance, cognitive slowing, and fatigue) and **hyperthyroidism** (tachycardia, body wasting, nervousness, tremor, and heat intolerance).

Drugs Used to Treat Hypothyroidism

Triidothyronine, levothyroxine

Mechanism of Action—*Triidothyronine* is T3, and *levothyroxine* is T4, which is converted to T3 at target tissues.

- T3 is the physiologically active hormone at target tissues.

Side Effects—Nervousness, tachycardia, heat intolerance, weight loss

Drugs Used to Treat Hyperthyroidism

Radioactive iodine, propylthiouracil (PTU), methimazole, iodide

RADIOACTIVE IODINE

Mechanism of Action—Thyroid follicular cells selectively uptake radioactive iodine (^{131}I). Radioactive iodine emits beta particles, resulting in the **destruction of thyroid follicular cells** and alleviation of hyperthyroidism.

Side Effects—Hypothyroidism is common, requiring the patient to take *levothyroxine*.

HARDCORE

Octreotide is the synthetic analog of *somatostatin*.

HARDCORE

When administered in **pulsatile** fashion, leuprolide increases GnRH release and results in subsequent ovulation. When administered **continuously**, leuprolide suppresses the production of gonadal hormones (LH and FSH) and can be used to treat prostate cancer, endometriosis, and uterine fibroids.

HARDCORE

Uterine sensitivity to *oxytocin* increases with the duration of pregnancy.

HARDCORE

Vasopressin also activates V-1 receptors in vascular smooth muscle, which may cause headache, bronchoconstriction, and tremor. *Desmopressin* does not act on the V-1 receptor, therefore does not have any pressor side effects.

HARDCORE

Vasopressin can be dangerous in patients with CAD, CHF, asthma, and epilepsy.

HARDCORE

Levothyroxine has a long half-life, and steady state is not achieved until 6 to 8 weeks after onset of therapy.

HARDCORE

Levothyroxine and *triidothyronine* have the same efficacy, but *levothyroxine* is used clinically because it is much cheaper and requires less frequent administration than *liothyronine*.

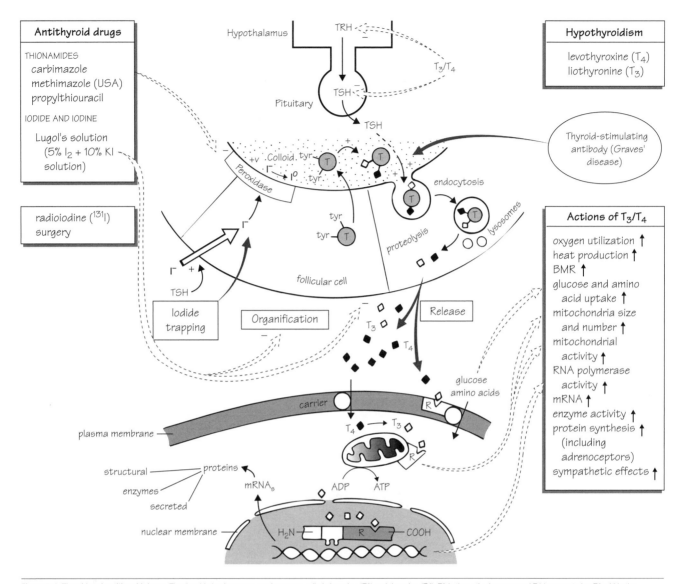

Figure 7-4 Thyroid and antithyroid drugs. The thyroid gland secretes two hormones, triiodothyronine (T3) and thyroxine (T4). T3 is the active hormone and T4 is converted to T3 within the periphery. Synthesis of T3 and T4 in thyroid follicular cells requires iodine. Iodine is first concentrated in the cell, where it is then oxidized by peroxidase to a more reactive form. Iodine then reacts with tyrosine residues present in thyroglobulin, a process called organification, forming units of T3 and T4. The subsequent release of thyroid hormone is regulated by thyroid stimulating hormone (TSH), which is released from the anterior pituitary gland in response to reduced levels of circulating thyroid hormone. (Reprinted with permission from Neal MJ. Medical Pharmacology at a Glance. 4th ed. Oxford: Blackwell Publishing, 2002:76.)

METHIMAZOLE

Mechanism of Action—Inhibits thyroid hormone synthesis by:

- *Inhibiting the oxidative process* required for iodination of tyrosyl groups
- *Preventing the coupling* of iodotyrosines that form T3 and T4

Side Effects—Agranulocytosis, rash, edema

PROPYLTHIOURACIL (PTU)

Mechanism of Action—Inhibits thyroid hormone synthesis by:

- *Inhibiting the oxidative process* required for iodination of tyrosyl groups
- *Preventing the coupling* of iodotyrosines that form T3 and T4
- *Blocking the peripheral conversion* of T4 to T3

Side Effects—Agranulocytosis, rash, edema

IODIDE

Indications and Usage—Prior to neck/thyroid surgery (decreases thyroid gland vascularity) and in thyroid storm (emergently)

Mechanism of Action—*Inhibits the iodination of tyrosine* to decrease the supply of stored thyroglobulin; *inhibits release of stored thyroid hormone*

Side Effects—Sore mouth and throat, rashes, mucous membrane ulcerations

HARDCORE

Both *methimazole* and *PTU* are slow in onset and, therefore, are not effective in the treatment of thyroid storm.

HARDCORE

After several weeks, the thyroid gland will not respond to iodide treatment, so this agent is only used in short-term therapy.

HARDCORE REVIEW – ENDOCRINE PHARMACOLOGY

TABLE 7-2	Drugs Used to Treat Diabetes Mellitus		
DRUG CLASS	**DRUGS**	**MECHANISM OF ACTION**	**MAJOR SIDE EFFECTS**
Insulin	Regular—rapid	Phosphorylation of tyrosine kinase	Hypoglycemia
	Lispro—most rapid		
	Semilente—intermediate		
	NPH—intermediate		
	Lente—intermediate		
	Ultralente—long acting		
	Insulin glargine—longest acting		
Sulfonylureas	First generation: Tolbutamide Chlorpropamide	Increase pancreatic release of insulin and improve tissue sensitivity	Hypoglycemia
	Second generation: Glyburide Glipizide		
Biguanide	Metformin	Inhibits hepatic gluconeogenesis	Lactic acidosis
Glitazones	Rosiglitazone, pioglitazone	Improve tissue sensitivity	Weight gain, hepatotoxicity
α-Glucosidase inhibitor	Acarbose	Inhibits α-glucosidase	Flatulence

TABLE 7-3	Steroid Hormones		
DRUG CLASS	**DRUGS**	**MECHANISM OF ACTION**	**MAJOR SIDE EFFECTS**
Estrogens	Estradiol, estriol, estrone, ethinyl estradiol, DES	Bind estrogen receptors	Venous thromboembolism
Antiestrogens	Clomiphene	Block estrogen negative feedback	Ovarian enlargement, vasomotor flushes
	Tamoxifen, raloxifene	Compete for estrogen receptors	Hot flashes, vaginal bleeding
Progestins	Medroxyprogesterone, hydroxyprogesterone, norethindrone, norgestrel	Bind progesterone receptors	Edema, depression, increase LDL levels
Antiprogestins	Mifepristone	Decrease hCG	Uterine bleeding
Androgens	Testosterone, danazol, nandrolone, stanozolol, fluoxymesterone	Bind testosterone receptors	Masculinization, priapism, impotence
Antiandrogens	Finasteride	Inhibits 5-α-reductase, decreases DHT levels	Feminization
	Flutamide Ketoconazole/ spironolactone	Competitive inhibitor Inhibits steroid synthesis	Feminization Pruritus, hair loss, hemolytic anemia

TABLE 7-4 Corticosteroids

Drug Class	Drugs	Mechanism of Action	Major Side Effects
Glucocorticoids	*Hydrocortisone, cortisone, prednisone, prednisolone, methylprednisone, betamethasone, dexamethasone*	Induce transcription factors, inhibit phospholipase A2	Cushing-like syndrome (truncal obesity, buffalo hump, moon facies, acne, insomnia), osteoporosis, infection, hyperglycemia
Mineralocorticoids	*Fludrocortisone deoxycorticosterone*	Induce transcription factors, inhibit phospholipase A_2	Cushing-like syndrome

TABLE 7-5 Drugs Used to Treat Osteoporosis

Drug Class	Drugs	Mechanism of Action	Major Side Effects
Bisphosphonates	*Alendronate, pamidronate, risedronate*	Inhibit osteoclast activity	Erosive esophageal damage
Calcium carbonate	*Calcium carbonate*	Supplementation	GI discomfort
Calcitonin	*Calcitonin*	Inhibits osteoclasts	Flushing, nausea
Hormone replacement therapy	*Estrogen*	Inhibits osteoclasts	Risk of heart attack, stroke, deep vein thrombosis, pulmonary emboli, breast cancer

TABLE 7-6 Hormones of the Pituitary Gland

Drug Class	Drugs	Mechanism of Action	Major Side Effects
Somatostatin analogs	*Somatostatin, octreotide*	Hormone inhibitor	Flatulence, steatorrhea
GnRH antagonists	*Leuprolide*	GnRH antagonist	Antiandrogen
Oxytocin	*Oxytocin*	Uterine contractions	Water retention
ADH	*Vasopressin, desmopressin*	Increase water resorption	Water intoxication, hyponatremia

TABLE 7-7 Thyroid Hormones

Drug Class	Drugs	Mechanism of Action	Major Side Effects
Treatment of hypothyroidism	*Levothyroxine*	T4 hormone	Nervousness, tachycardia
	Triiodothyronine	T3 hormone	Nervousness, tachycardia
Treatment of hyperthyroidism	*Radioactive iodine*	Emits beta particles	Hypothyroidism
	Methimazole	Inhibits oxidation and coupling	Agranulocytosis
	PTU	Inhibits oxidation, coupling and T4 to T3 conversion	Agranulocytosis
	Iodide	Inhibits iodination and thyroid hormone release	Mucous membrane ulcerations

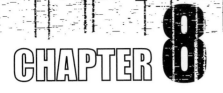

CHAPTER 8

Gastrointestinal Pharmacology

Gastrointestinal (GI) function is regulated by a number of endogenous compounds. These compounds control GI contraction and relaxation, the secretion of digestive enzymes, and the secretion of fluid and electrolytes. Table 8-1 lists the major endogenous compounds that act on the GI tract.

The hormones and neurotransmitters listed in Table 8-1 can be manipulated pharmacologically to treat gastrointestinal medical conditions, including peptic ulcer disease, gastroesophageal reflux disease, diarrhea, constipation, and emesis.

DRUGS USED TO TREAT PEPTIC ULCER DISEASE AND GASTROESOPHAGEAL REFLUX DISEASE

Drugs used to eradicate *Helicobacter pylori*—*Bismuth, metronidazole, tetracycline, amoxicillin*

Histamine receptor blockers—*Cimetidine, famotidine, ranitidine, nizatidine*

Proton pump inhibitors (PPIs)—*Omeprazole and lansoprazole*

Antacids—*Aluminum hydroxide, magnesium hydroxide, calcium carbonate*

Cytoprotective agents—*Sucralfate, misoprostol*

A peptic ulcer is a mucosal break that can involve the stomach or duodenum. Some of the most common contributing factors are the presence of *H. pylori*, overuse of NSAIDs, and excessive acid secretion. The term peptic ulcer disease (PUD) generally refers to a spectrum of disorders, including gastric ulcers, pyloric channel ulcers, duodenal ulcers, and postoperative ulcers.

Gastroesophageal reflux is a normal physiologic event experienced occasionally by most people, particularly after a meal. Gastroesophageal reflux disease (GERD) occurs when the amount of gastric juice that refluxes into the esophagus is excessive and results in esophageal mucosal injury (esophagitis). Lower esophageal sphincter relaxation secondary to a hiatal hernia is one of the most common causes.

TABLE 8-1	Major Endogenous Regulators of GI Function		
Endogenous Compound	**Site of Secretion**	**Secretory Stimulus**	**Action(s) on the GI Tract**
Acetylcholine	Cholinergic neurons	• Stimulation of the parasympathetic nervous system	• Contraction of GI smooth muscle • Relaxation of sphincters • Increased gastric and pancreatic secretions
Norepinephrine	Adrenergic neurons	• Stimulation of the sympathetic nervous system	• Relaxation of GI smooth muscle • Contraction of sphincters
Gastrin	Stomach G cells	• Vagal stimulation • Stomach distention • Peptides	• Increased gastric H^+ secretion
Pepsin	Stomach chief cells	• Local acid • Vagal stimulation	• Digestion of protein
Secretin	Duodenal S cells	• Acid in duodenum • Fatty acids in the duodenum	• Increased bicarbonate secretion • Decreased gastric acid secretion
Somatostatin	δ cells of the islets of Langerhans	• Ingestion of nutrients (glucose, amino acids, fatty acids) • Glucagon	• Inhibition of insulin and glucagon secretion
Cholecystokinin	Duodenal and jejunal I cells	• Fatty acids • Amino acids	• Increased pancreatic enzyme and bicarbonate secretion • Inhibition of gastric emptying • Gallbladder contraction

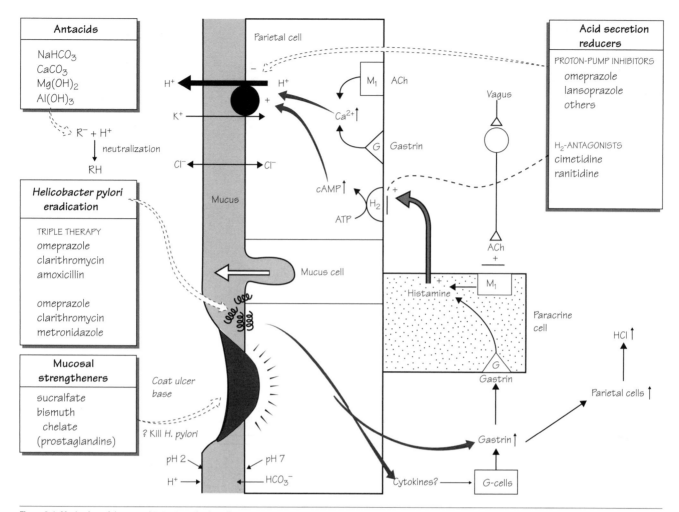

Figure 8-1 Mechanism of drugs used to treat peptic ulcer disease and reduce gastric acid secretion. (Reprinted with permission from Neal MJ. Medical Pharmacology at a Glance. 4th ed. Oxford: Blackwell Publishing, 2002:30.)

The treatment of PUD and GERD is directed at restoring the physiologic balance between gastric acid secretion and mucosal protection to limit erosion of the gastric lining. In addition, it is now clear that *H. pylori* infection is one of the primary contributing mechanisms in the development of PUD (duodenal), and therefore the eradication of the gram-negative *H. pylori* is essential for management of these patients.

Drugs Used to Eradicate *H. pylori*

Eradication of *H. pylori* typically consists of triple therapy, including:

1. *Bismuth*
2. *Metronidazole*
3. Either *tetracycline or amoxicillin*

These drugs are covered in detail in the following sections (*bismuth*) and in Chapter 10.

Histamine Receptor Blockers

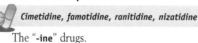 *Cimetidine, famotidine, ranitidine, nizatidine*

The "**-ine**" drugs.

Indications and Usage—PUD, GERD, Zollinger-Ellison syndrome, acute stress ulcers, gastritis

Mechanism of Action—Block **histamine H₂-receptors**, resulting in a decrease in gastric acid secretion

Side Effects—Side effects are primarily associated with the agent **cimetidine** and include:

- **Inhibition of P-450**, slowing the metabolism of several drugs including *warfarin, phenytoin, quinidine, carbamazepine, theophylline,* and *imipramine*. Consequently, blood levels of these drugs will be **higher than expected** when administered concurrently with *cimetidine*.

- Antiandrogenic effects, leading to **gynecomastia** and **galactorrhea**

- CNS effects in the elderly, including confusion and hallucinations

- Headaches, dizziness, and diarrhea

HARDCORE

Histamine receptor blockers are **competitive antagonists and reversible**, in contrast to proton-pump inhibitors (*omeprazole*), which are irreversible.

Proton Pump Inhibitors

Omeprazole, lansoprazole

The "**-prazole**" drugs, "the *-ole* pump inhibitors."

Indications and Usage—PUD, GERD, Zollinger-Ellison syndrome, erosive esophagitis

Mechanism of Action—Binds to the **H^+/K^+-ATPase pump in parietal cells**, suppressing the secretion of hydrogen ions into the gastric lumen. Recall that any compounds that stimulate gastric acid secretion (i.e., gastrin, histamine, and acetylcholine) require the action of this proton pump to secrete H^+ into the stomach lumen. Therefore, inhibiting the H^+/K^+-ATPase pump is effective in reducing the secretion of gastric acid.

Side Effects—Diarrhea and dizziness. Additionally, *omeprazole* interferes with the oxidation of *warfarin, phenytoin, diazepam,* and *cyclosporine,* resulting in increased blood levels of these drugs if used concurrently.

Antacids

Aluminum hydroxide, magnesium hydroxide, calcium carbonate

Indications and Usage—GERD, promotion of duodenal ulcer healing

Mechanism of Action—These agents are **weak bases** capable of neutralizing gastric acid.

Side Effects—Chelation and decreased absorption of certain drugs such as the *tetracycline antibiotics and levodopa*

Cytoprotective Agents

Sucralfate, misoprostol

SUCRALFATE

Indications and Usage—*PUD*

Mechanism of Action—Interacts with the gastric mucosa to form a **complex gel**, creating a physical barrier that impairs the diffusion of HCl and prevents pepsin-mediated degradation of mucosa

Side Effects—Nausea, decreased absorption of other oral drugs taken concurrently

HARDCORE

The effects of proton pump inhibitors are longer lasting than H₂-blockers, because they ***irreversibly*** inhibit the proton pump. For the parietal cells to overcome this inhibition, they must synthesize entirely new H⁺/K⁺-ATPase proteins.

HARDCORE

In older patients, PPIs greatly increase the risk of **Campylobacter *infection***, because they eliminate the body's natural defense of a highly acidic gastric environment.

HARDCORE

Overuse of aluminum-containing antacids can cause constipation, whereas the overuse of magnesium-containing antacids can cause diarrhea.

HARDCORE

Calcium salts stimulate gastrin release, so calcium-containing antacids may lead to rebound hyperacidity.

HARDCORE

The hormone ***pepsin*** functions optimally at a pH of 1.0–3.0 to digest proteins. Because antacids increase gastric pH, they can reduce pepsin activity.

HARDCORE

Sucralfate ***requires an acidic pH for activation***, so it should not be administered with H₂ antagonists or antacids.

HARDCORE

Sucralfate combines with and limits the absorption of *tetracyclines, cimetidine, digoxin,* and *phenytoin*.

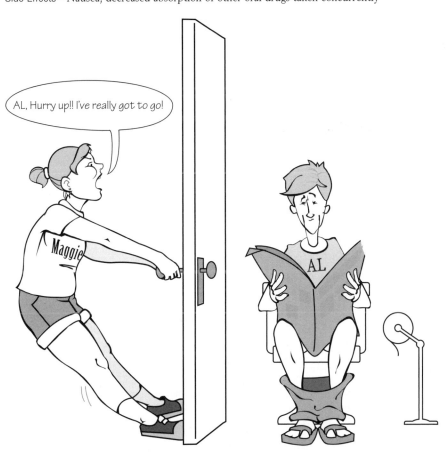

AL, Hurry up!! I've really got to go!

Figure 8-2 **AL** had too much **AL**uminum and can't go – **MAG**gie had too much **MAG**nesium and can't wait to go.

Misoprostol and other PGE$_1$ analogs produce **uterine contractions** and are contraindicated in pregnant women.

MISOPROSTOL

Indications and Usage—PUD, patients at high risk for NSAID-induced ulcers

Mechanism of Action—Misoprostol is a prostaglandin E$_1$ analog. Prostaglandins (normally produced by the gastric mucosa) inhibit the secretion of HCl from parietal cells and stimulate the secretion of mucus and bicarbonate.

Side Effects—Diarrhea and nausea

DRUGS USED TO TREAT DIARRHEA

Antimotility drugs are analogs of the opioid *meperidine*.

- **LO**peramide is used for diarrhea – s**LO**w the f**LO**w!

These agents may cause **toxic megacolon** in children or patients with severe colitis.

Because *loperamide* does not cross the blood-brain barrier, it will not produce the euphoria or respiratory depression characteristic of other opioids.

> **Antimotility drugs:** *Diphenoxylate, loperamide*
> **Adsorbants:** *Kaolin, pectin, methylcellulose*

Agents that relieve diarrhea act by altering intestinal motility and slowing transit time in the GI tract, or by increasing stool viscosity.

Antimotility Drugs

> *Diphenoxylate, loperamide*

Mechanism of Action—Activate **presynaptic opioid receptors in the enteric nervous system**, inhibiting peristalsis and prolonging fecal transit time

Side Effects—Drowsiness, abdominal cramps, dizziness

Adsorbants

> *Kaolin, pectin, methylcellulose*

Mechanism of Action—**Adsorbs intestinal toxins and microorganisms**, protecting the intestinal mucosa and increasing stool viscosity

Side Effects—These agents can interfere with the absorption of other oral drugs taken concurrently.

DRUGS USED TO TREAT CONSTIPATION

Constipation is the abnormally delayed or infrequent passage of dry, hardened feces. Laxatives are drugs used to relieve constipation. There are three categories of laxatives: **stool softeners, stimulants (irritants)**, and **bulking agents**. Remember that in most cases, excluding hospitalized patients, constipation can usually be treated nonpharmacologically by increasing intake of water and dietary fiber.

Stool Softeners

> *Mineral oil, glycerin, docusate*

Mechanism of Action—These agents create a **hyperosmotic** environment, which draws water into the lumen of the intestines. Additionally, they lubricate the feces to ease intestinal transit.

Side Effects—Cramps, diarrhea, and flatulence

Stimulants

> *Phenolphthalein, bisacodyl, castor oil, senna*

Mechanism of Action—**Irritate the mucosal lining**, inducing hypermotility of the intestines and their contents

Side Effects—If used chronically, these agents can cause rebound intestinal hypomotility when discontinued.

If used for prolonged periods, *senna and castor oil* can irritate intestinal nerves.

Bulking Agents

> *Psyllium, methylcellulose*

Mechanism of Action—These agents contain nondigestable plant products, creating a hyperosmotic environment that draws water into the intestinal lumen, making the transit of GI contents smoother.

Side Effects—Flatulence

DRUGS USED TO TREAT EMESIS

Phenothiazines: *Prochlorperazine*

Substituted benzamide: *Metoclopramide*

Cannabinoids: *Dronabinol, nabilone*

5-HT₃ serotonin receptor blockers: *Granisetron, ondansetron*

Emesis is a poorly understood process involving complex interactions with multiple neuronal structures and receptors. The vomiting center in the brain receives major inputs from the gut, the cardiovascular system, the limbic brain nuclei, and the chemoreceptor trigger zone (CTZ). The CTZ is a circumventricular organ located at the caudal end of the fourth ventricle (area postrema) that lacks an effective blood-brain barrier, and responds to emetogenic agents in the systemic circulation by initiating the vomit reflex. Most agents used to treat emesis act by blocking specific neurotransmitter receptor sites within the vomiting circuit including dopamine, serotonin, muscarinic, histamine, and substance P receptors.

Phenothiazines

Prochlorperazine

Mechanism of Action—***Blocks mesolimbic dopaminergic D₁ and D₂ receptors*** in the medullary CTZ

Side Effects—Extrapyramidal symptoms (EPS), including Parkinsonian symptoms and motor restlessness; sedation

Substituted Benzamides

Metoclopramide

Mechanism of Action—***Blocks dopamine and serotonin receptors in the CTZ***. Also enhances gut motility and accelerates gastric emptying without stimulating gastric, biliary, or pancreatic secretions

Side Effects—Sedation, diarrhea, EPS

Cannabinoids

Dronabinol, nabilone

Mechanism of Action—Unknown, (likely involves anandamide receptors)

Side Effects—Sedation, vertigo, disorientation

5-HT₃ Serotonin Receptor Blockers

Granisetron, ondansetron

Mechanism of Action—Selective ***blockade of 5-HT₃ receptors*** in the CTZ

Side Effects—Headache

HARDCORE

Cannabinoid antiemetic action may actually not involve the brain, because synthetic cannabinoids *lack psychotrophic activity* (unlike the classic cannabinoid *cannabis*).

HARDCORE

Cannabinoids are effective in treating chemotherapy-induced emesis.

HARDCORE

Recall that drugs used to treat migraine (e.g., *sumatriptan*) are 5-HT agonists. Therefore, caution should be used when treating migraine-prone patients with 5-HT antagonists.

HARDCORE REVIEW—GASTROINTESTINAL PHARMACOLOGY

TABLE 8-2 Drugs Used to Treat PUD and GERD

Drug Class	Drugs	Mechanism of Action	Major Side Effects
Histamine receptor blockers	*Cimetidine, famotidine, ranitidine, nizatidine*	Parietal cell H₂-receptor blocker	*Cimetidine*: P-450 inhibition, gynecomastia and decreased renal creatinine clearance
Proton-pump inhibitors	*Omeprazole, lansoprazole*	H⁺/K⁺-ATPase proton pump inhibitor	Drug interactions
Antacids	*Aluminum hydroxide, magnesium hydroxide, calcium carbonate*	Neutralize gastric acid	Drug interactions, diarrhea, constipation
Prostaglandins	*Misoprostol*	Stimulate the secretion of mucus and bicarbonate	Uterine contractions, contraindicated in pregnancy
Mucosal protective agents	*Sucralfate*	Create a barrier that prevents degradation of mucus by pepsin	Nausea

TABLE 8-3 Drugs Used to Treat Diarrhea

Drug Class	Drugs	Mechanism of Action	Major Side Effects
Antimotility drugs	*Diphenoxylate, loperamide*	Activate opioid receptors that decrease peristalsis	Drowsiness, cramps, toxic megacolon
Adsorbants	*Kaolin, pectin, methylcellulose*	Adsorption of intestinal toxins, mucosal protection	Interfere with drug absorption

TABLE 8-4 Drugs Used to Treat Constipation

Drug Class	Drugs	Mechanism of Action	Major Side Effects
Stool softeners	*Mineral oil, glycerin, docusate*	Hyperosmotic agents	GI discomfort
Stimulants/irritants	*Phenolphthalein, bisacodyl, castor oil, senna*	Mucosal lining irritants	Rebound intestinal hypomotility
Bulking agents	*Psyllium, methylcellulose*	Draws water into intestinal lumen	Flatulence

TABLE 8-5 Drugs Used to Treat Emesis

Drug Class	Drugs	Mechanism of Action	Major Side Effects
Phenothiazines	*Prochlorperazine*	Block dopamine receptors	EPS
Substituted benzamides	*Metoclopramide*	Block dopamine receptors	EPS
Cannabinoids	*Dronabinol, nabilone*	G-protein agonist	Dysphoria, hallucinations
5-HT$_3$ serotonin receptor blockers	*Granisetron, ondansetron*	Block 5-HT$_3$ receptors	Headache

CHAPTER 9

Chemotherapeutics and Immunomodulator Pharmacology

The term *cancer* refers to a pathologic state in which cellular mutations cause abnormally rapid tissue growth. Cancer can develop in almost any type of tissue and varies widely in its prognostic course. Although treatment of cancer can include chemotherapy, radiation, and surgery, the board exam will expect you to be familiar with only chemotherapeutic agents. Indications for specific chemotherapeutic treatment regimens are constantly being altered and upgraded, so outside of a few classic cancers, the board exam will focus on the differences in the mechanisms of action and side effects between the major drugs and classes of drugs.

 Alkylating agents: *Cisplatin, carboplatin, cyclophosphamide, chlorambucil, streptozocin, carmustine, busulfan*

Antimetabolites: *Methotrexate, 6-mercaptopurine (6MP), fluorouracil (5-FU), capecitabine, cytarabine (ara-C), 6-thioguanine*

Antibiotics: *Bleomycin, dactinomycin, actinomycin, mitomycin C, doxorubicin (Adriamycin), daunorubicin*

Microtubule inhibitors (Vinca alkaloids/taxols): *Vincristine, vinblastine, paclitaxel, docetaxel*

Topoisomerase inhibitors: *Topotecan, etoposide*

Hormonal agents: *Tamoxifen, flutamide, leuprolide, anastrozole*

Monoclonal antibodies: *Rituximab, imiximab*

Immunosuppressants: *Azathioprine, mycophenolate, cyclosporine, tacrolimus (FK506), muromonab-CD3 (OKT3)*

DRUGS USED TO TREAT CANCER

Alkylating Agents

Cisplatin, carboplatin, mechlorethamine, cyclophosphamide, chlorambucil, streptozocin, busulfan

These agents covalently bind to various cell constituents, including DNA. **DNA alkylation interferes with DNA synthesis and is lethal to the cell.**

CISPLATIN AND CARBOPLATIN (PLATINUM ANALOGS)

Indications—Cancers of the testes, ovaries, cervix, bladder, and lung

Mechanism of Action—Forms **cross-links in DNA** that interfere with DNA function and replication

Side Effects

- *Cisplatin*: **Neuropathy** (e.g., paresthesias), **nephropathy**, **ototoxicity**, myelosuppression, severe nausea/vomiting
- *Carboplatin*: **Myelosuppression**, thrombocytopenia, leukopenia

MECHLORETHAMINE AND CYCLOPHOSPHAMIDE (NITROGEN MUSTARDS)

Indications—Lymphomas, leukemia (cyclophosphamide), breast cancers

Mechanism of Action—Form **cross-links in DNA** that interfere with DNA function and replication. These drugs **do not differentiate between resting and cycling cells**.

Side Effects

- *Mechlorethamine*: Myelosuppression, skin rash
- *Cyclophosphamide*: **Hemorrhagic cystitis**, inappropriate release of ADH (SIADH), myelosuppression, alopecia

HARDCORE

The platinum analogs are considered cell cycle-nonspecific but work best in cells that are rapidly multiplying.

HARDCORE

*Carboplatin is **not** associated with nephro-, oto-, or neurotoxicity.*

HARDCORE

With **CIS**platin you may not be able to **piss** (nephropathy), you will **miss** what others are saying (ototoxicity), and won't feel the **kiss** (neuropathy) of your mate, **suppressing** the desire of **Myelo S.** to date you (myelosuppression).

HARDCORE

Cyclophosphamide-induced hemorrhagic cystitis can be treated clinically with **hydration and mensa**, an antidote that binds and helps excrete the urotoxic metabolite of *cyclophosphamide*.

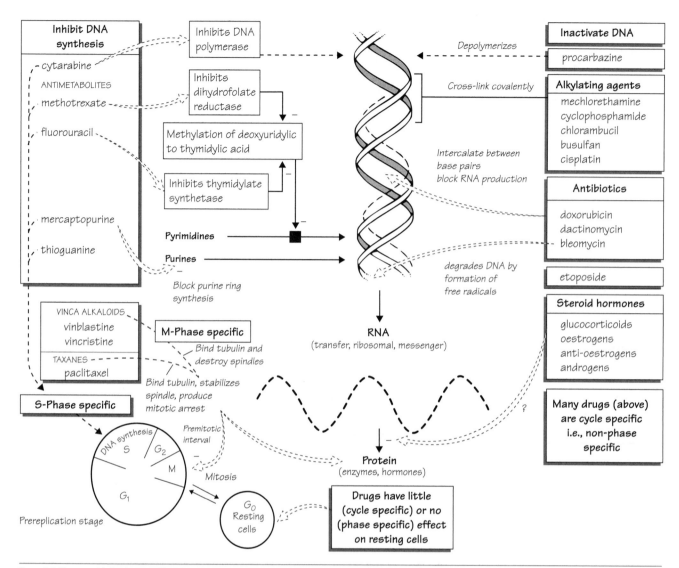

Figure 9-1 Drugs used to treat cancer. Chemotherapeutics act by inhibiting the mechanisms of cell proliferation, and therefore are toxic to both tumor cells and normal rapidly proliferating cells. Chemotherapuetics are classified according to their sites of action. Some drugs are only effective during part of the cell cycle (cell cycle-specific) while others are cytotoxic throughout the cell cycle (cell cycle-nonspecific). (Reprinted with permission from Neal MJ. Medical Pharmacology at a Glance. 4th ed. Oxford: Blackwell Publishing, 2002:92.)

HARDCORE

Lipid-soluble drugs, like the nitrosoureas, are important for the treatment of *brain tumors*, because they are capable of achieving high concentrations in the CNS.

CARMUSTINE AND STREPTOZOCIN (NITROSOUREAS)

Indications—Lymphomas, brain tumors, pancreatic insulinomas

Mechanism of Action—Form cross-links in DNA that interfere with DNA function and replication. These drugs *do not differentiate between resting and cycling cells*.

Side Effects—Myelosuppression, also renal toxicity and *pulmonary fibrosis* if used chronically

BUSULFAN

Indications—Chronic myelogenous leukemia (CML) and marrow ablation prior to bone marrow transplant in patients with myeloid cancers (e.g., multiple myeloma, AML, etc.)

Mechanism of Action—Form cross-links in DNA that interfere with DNA function and replication. These drugs *do not differentiate between resting and cycling cells*.

Side Effects—Myelosuppression, *pulmonary fibrosis*, hyperpigmentation

Antimetabolites

Methotrexate, 6MP, 6-thioguanine, 5-FU, ara-C

METHOTREXATE (FOLATE ANTAGONIST)

Indications—Leukemia, lymphoma, sarcoma, breast cancer

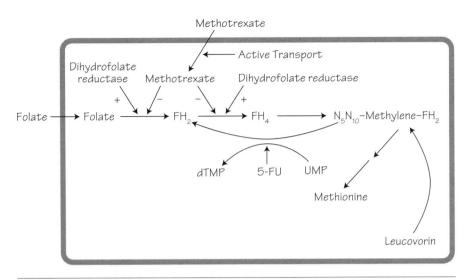

Figure 9-2 Intracellular mechanism of methotrexate with leucovorin rescue. *Leucovorin* is a reduced form of folate that does not require the use of DHFR, and is capable of resupplying cells with the necessary folate for DNA and RNA synthesis. *Leucovorin* is taken up more readily by normal cells than tumor cells (because tumor cells have impaired transport mechanisms), and essentially "***rescues***" normal body tissues from the severe toxicity associated with methotrexate use. This is referred to as the "***leucovorin rescue.***"

Mechanism of Action—Inhibits ***dihydrofolate reductase***, the enzyme responsible for the conversion of folate into dihydrofolic acid (folate reduction). Inhibition of dihydrofolate reductase results in ***reduced synthesis of the purines, thymidylate, serine, and methionine*** necessary for DNA and RNA synthesis.

Side Effects—Myelosuppression, hepatotoxicity, stomatitis, mucositis, renal dysfunction

- Think of a **T-Rex** (*metho***TREX***ate*) with bleeding gums (*mucositis*), after feasting on the liver (*hepatotoxicity*) and kidneys (*renal dysfunction*), and sucking the bones dry (*myelosuppression*) of a Scared (*S phase*) dinosaur

6-MERCAPTOPURINE AND 6-THIOGUANINE (PURINE ANTIMETABOLITE)

Indications—Leukemia

Mechanism of Action—These agents are metabolized into ***false purine analogs***, which inhibit enzymes involved in purine interconversion, resulting in cytotoxicity.

Side Effects—***Neutropenia***, rash

- *Mercapto*purine **captures** neutrophils from circulation, resulting in neutropenia.

5-FLUOROURACIL AND CAPECITABINE (PYRIMIDINE ANTIMETABOLITE)

Indications

- *5-Fluorouracil*: Main use is for gastrointestinal malignancies (gastric, colon, and rectal cancers); breast and bladder cancers
- *Capecitabine*: Metastatic breast cancer

Mechanism of Action—These agents are metabolized into ***false pyrimidine analogs***, which act by inhibiting synthesis of thymidine and by incorporating into cellular RNA. The effects on DNA and RNA result in cytotoxicity.

Side Effects—Stomatitis, severe diarrhea, rash, alopecia, hyperpigmentation, myelosuppression, and ***neurotoxicity***

CYTARABINE (ARA-C; PYRIMIDINE ANTAGONIST)

Indications—Acute myelogenous leukemia

Mechanism of Action—Acts as a ***competitive antagonist of DNA polymerase***. It can also be incorporated into DNA and RNA, resulting in termination of chain elongation.

Side Effects—Myelosuppression (primarily ***granulocytopenia***), hepatic dysfunction, seizures

Antibiotics

Bleomycin, ***dactinomycin, actinomycin, mitomycin C,*** doxorubicin **(Adriamycin),** *daunorubicin*

These agents are termed "antibiotics" because they are natural products derived from the bacterial species *Streptomyces*.

HARDCORE

Methotrexate is cell cycle-specific for the ***S phase***.

HARDCORE

Treatment with *methotrexate* is typically followed by administration of *leucovorin*, a reduced form of folate that does not require the use of DHFR. *Leucovorin* is taken up more readily by normal cells than tumor cells (because tumor cells have impaired transport mechanisms), and essentially "***rescues***" normal body tissues from the severe toxicity associated with methotrexate use. This is referred to as the "***leucovorin rescue.***" (see Figure 9-2).

HARDCORE

Ara-C is **S-phase** specific; it works in the cell cycle.

HARDCORE

Bleomycin is cell cycle-specific: *Blocks at G2*.

BLEOMYCIN

Indications—Testicular cancer, lymphoma

Mechanism of Action—Forms a *ferrous iron-oxygen drug complex* that cleaves DNA

Side Effects—*Pulmonary fibrosis*, pneumonitis, Raynaud's phenomenon

DACTINOMYCIN AND ACTINOMYCIN

Indications—Soft tissue sarcoma, neuroblastoma

Mechanism of Action—Binds tightly to DNA and intercalates between base pairs, resulting in inhibition of DNA-dependent RNA synthesis and, ultimately, protein synthesis

Side Effects—Alopecia, myelosuppression

MITOMYCIN C

Indications—Bladder cancer

Mechanism of Action—Metabolically activated to an alkylating agent that cross-links DNA; generation of reactive oxygen radicals that damage DNA may also occur

Side Effects—Severe myelosuppression, *interstitial pneumonitis, nephrotoxicity*

HARDCORE

Doxorubicin may cause an *irreversible cardiomyopathy* syndrome that presents as congestive heart failure.

- Remember: **Adria**n (*adria*mycin) and **Rubi**n (*doxo*rubicin and *dauno*rubicin*) were two lovers who **married** (*intercalate DNA base pairs*) after Adrian **suppressed** (*myelosuppression*) Rubin's **alopecia** by **blocking** (*inhibiting*) him from wearing his **top** hat (*topoisomerase*).

DOXORUBICIN (ADRIAMYCIN)/DAUNORUBICIN

Indications—Solid tumors (sarcomas and adenocarcinomas) and hematologic malignancies (leukemia, lymphoma, multiple myeloma)

Mechanism of Action—Intercalate between DNA base pairs, interfering with DNA-dependent RNA synthesis; inhibition of DNA topoisomerases I and II, resulting in DNA strand breaks; generation of free radicals

Side Effects—*Cardiotoxicity*, including arrhythmias and delayed cardiomyopathy; myelosuppression; alopecia; mucositis

Microtubule Inhibitors

Vinca alkaloids: *Vincristine, vinblastine*
Taxols: *Paclitaxel, docetaxel*

VINCA ALKALOIDS

Vincristine, vinblastine, vinorelbine

HARDCORE

Vincristine, vinblastine, and vinorelbine are cell cycle-specific for the *M phase*.

Indications

- *Vincristine*: Leukemia, sarcoma, lymphoma
- *Vinblastine*: Lymphoma; testicular and renal cancers
- *Vinorelbine*: Lung, breast, and ovarian cancers; lymphoma

HARDCORE

Vinblastine is associated with *myelosuppression* (neutropenia and thrombocytopenia).

- Vin**BLAST**ine **blasts** away the marrow, causing myelosuppression.

Mechanism of Action—*Inhibit the polymerization of tubulin*, which is necessary for the formation of mitotic spindles for mitosis

Side Effects—Peripheral neuropathy, ileus

TAXOLS

Paclitaxel, docetaxel

HARDCORE

Paclitaxel and docetaxel are cell cycle-specific for the *G2 and M phases*.

Indications—Ovarian carcinoma, node-positive breast cancer, non-small cell lung cancer, AIDS-related Kaposi's sarcoma

Mechanism of Action—*Binds to tubulin and stabilizes microtubules*. The stabilized microtubules are dysfunctional and result in cell death.

Side Effects—Myelosuppression, *hepatic toxicity*, peripheral neuropathy, hypersensitivity reaction

Topoisomerase Inhibitors

Topotecan, etoposide

HARDCORE

Paclitaxel and docetaxel may also cause chromosome breakage by distorting the mitotic spindle apparatus.

Topoisomerases are nuclear enzymes that help maintain DNA in an appropriate state of supercoiling during replication. They are essential because, as DNA molecules uncoil during replication, torsion builds up within the DNA strands. Topoisomerases function by making cuts in the strands to relieve the strain placed on the DNA molecules. In addition, topoisomerases are able to repair the cuts they made following the completion of the replication.

Topotecan (Topoisomerase I Inhibitor)

Indications—Ovarian cancer, small cell and non-small cell lung cancer

Mechanism of Action—Inhibits **topoisomerase I**, which blocks replication and transcription

Side Effects—Myelosuppression, alopecia, fatigue, fever

HARDCORE

Topotecan is cell cycle-specific for the **late S** and **early G2** phases.

Etoposide (Topoisomerase II Inhibitor)

Indications—Small cell and non-small cell lung cancer, gastric cancer, germ cell cancers (e.g., testicular cancers), lymphoma, and leukemia

Mechanism of Action—Forms a **complex with topoisomerase II enzyme**, blocking DNA replication and causing DNA strand breakage

Side Effects—Myelosuppression, alopecia, stomatitis, skin changes

HARDCORE

Etoposide is cell cycle-specific for the **late S** and **early G2** phases.

Hormonal Agents

Antiestrogens: *Tamoxifen, raloxifene*

Antiandrogens: *Flutamide*

Aromatase inhibitors: *Anastrozole, letrozole*

Luteinizing hormone-releasing hormone (LHRH) agonists: *Leuprolide, goserelin*

Antiestrogens

Tamoxifen, raloxifene

Indications—Breast cancer (estrogen receptor [ER]-positive)

Mechanism of Action—*Tamoxifen* is a competitive partial agonist at estrogen receptors. Recall that a partial agonist (*tamoxifen*) can act as an antagonist in the presence of a full agonist (*estrogen*).

Side Effects—Hot flashes, mild nausea, vaginal dryness, hepatotoxicity, **endometrial cancer** (*tamoxifen*)

HARDCORE

In the breast, *tamoxifen* effectively antagonizes estrogen, but in the uterus it stimulates estrogen receptors and may lead to uterine hyperplasia and possibly cancer. *Raloxifene* also blocks breast estrogen receptors, but is not an agonist in the uterus.

Antiandrogens

Flutamide

Indications—Prostate cancer

Mechanism of Action—Inhibits androgen uptake and binding in target tissues

Side Effects—Hot flashes, **impotence**, gynecomastia

Aromatase Inhibitors

Anastrozole, letrozole

Indications—Breast cancer in postmenopausal women (ER-positive), usually reserved for patients who fail antiestrogen therapy

Mechanism of Action—**Inhibits the enzyme aromatase**, decreasing conversion of androgens to estrogen

Side Effects—Hot flashes, anorexia, edema

Leuprolide, goserelin

Indications—Prostate cancer, endometriosis

Mechanism of Action—These agents are gonadotropin releasing hormone (GnRH) receptor agonists, which suppress the production of luteinizing hormone (LH) and follicle-stimulating hormone (FSH), ultimately suppressing ovarian and testicular steroidogenesis

Side Effects—Hot flashes, weight gain, gynecomastia, depression

Monoclonal Antibodies

Rituximab, *imiximab*

Indication—B cell lymphoma

Mechanism of Action—Monoclonal antibody directed against the **CD20 surface antigen expressed on B-lymphocytes**

Side Effects—**Hypersensitivity**, leukopenia, thrombocytopenia

HARDCORE

Coating cancer cells with antibodies results in cell death by complement-mediated and antibody-dependent cell lysis, as well as the induction of apoptosis.

IMMUNOSUPPRESSANTS

 Azathioprine, mycophenolate, cyclosporine, tacrolimus (FK506), muromonab-CD3 (OKT3)

AZATHIOPRINE

Indications—Nonselective immunosuppression for organ transplantation

Mechanism of Action—An imidazolyl derivative of mercaptopurine, which is converted to 6-mercaptopurine (6-MP) in the body. **6-MP antagonizes purine metabolism, inhibiting the synthesis of DNA and RNA and, ultimately, proteins**.

Side Effects—Bone marrow depression, hepatotoxicity

MYCOPHENOLATE

Indications—Nonselective immunosuppression for organ transplantation

Mechanism of Action—Noncompetitive inhibitor of inosine monophosphate dehydrogenase that causes **blockade of the de novo formation of guanosine phosphate (GMP)**

Side Effects—Leukopenia, sepsis, lymphoma

CYCLOSPORINE

Indications—Selective immunosuppression for organ transplantation; rheumatoid arthritis

Mechanism of Action—Inhibits gene transcription of several factors produced by activated T cells, including IL-2

Side Effects—**Nephrotoxicity** (reversible), hepatotoxicity, infections, lymphoma, gingival hyperplasia

TACROLIMUS (FK506)

Indications—Selective immunosuppression for organ transplantation

Mechanism of Action—Diffuses into T cells, where it **binds FK binding protein (FKBP) resulting in inhibition of cytokine synthesis**

Side Effects—**Nephrotoxicity** and neurotoxicity, including seizures and hallucinations

MUROMONAB-CD3 (OKT3)

Indications—Acute rejection of renal, cardiac, or hepatic allografts

Mechanism of Action—OKT3 is a murine monoclonal antibody **directed against the CD3 molecule of human T cells**, resulting in blockade of antigen recognition and a decreased T cell-mediated immune response.

Side Effects—Anaphylaxis, seizures, encephalopathy, infections

HARDCORE REVIEW – CHEMOTHERAPEUTICS AND IMMUNOMODULATOR PHARMACOLOGY

Mechanisms of Genetic Resistance to Cytotoxic Drugs:

- Altered drug transport
- Increased expression of tumor cell genes
- Multidrug-resistance glycoprotein, which leads to efflux of drug by membrane protein
- Decreased cellular retention
- Increased cellular inactivation (both binding and metabolism)
- Altered target protein
- Enhanced repair of DNA damage
- Altered processing

HARDCORE

Lymphocytes are predominantly acted on by *azathioprine* due to their rapid proliferation required during the immune response and their dependence on *de novo* synthesis of purines for cell division.

HARDCORE

IL-2 stimulates further T lymphocyte production.

HARDCORE

Tacrolimus is 10 to 100 times more potent than *cyclosporine*.

HARDCORE

Muromonab is contraindicated in patients with a history of seizure and heart failure, as well as in pregnant and breast-feeding women.

TABLE 9-1	Chemotherapeutic Hardcore Side Effects
Myelosuppression	*Cyclophosphamide, busulfan, cisplatin, carboplatin, paclitaxel, methotrexate, cytarabine, etoposide, 6-mercaptopurine*
Non-myelosuppressive	*Vincristine, bleomycin*
Hemorrhagic cystitis	*Cyclophosphamide, ifosfamide*
Nephrotoxic	*Cisplatin, mitomycin C*
Pulmonary toxic	*Bleomycin, busulfan*
Cardiotoxic	*Doxorubicin, daunorubicin*
Neurotoxic	*Cisplatin, vincristine, paclitaxel*
Bladder cancer	*Cyclophosphamide*
Teratogenic	*Leflunomide, tamoxifen*
Allergy	*Paclitaxel*
Mouth ulcers	*Methotrexate*

TABLE 9-2	Alkylating Agents			
DRUG CLASS	**DRUGS**	**MECHANISM OF ACTION**	**HARDCORE CELL-CYCLE PHASE**	**MAJOR SIDE EFFECTS**
Alkylating Agents				*"All myelosuppress"*
Platinum analogs	**Cisplatin**	Cross-link DNA	Nonspecific	**Nephro-, oto-, neurotoxicities**
	Carboplatin	Cross-link DNA	Nonspecific	
Nitrogen mustards	**Cyclophosphamide**	Cross-link DNA	Nonspecific	**Hemorrhagic cystitis**, SIADH
	Mechlorethamine	Cross-link DNA	Nonspecific	
Nitrosoureas	*Carmustine*	Cross-link DNA	Nonspecific	
	Streptozocin	Cross-link DNA	Nonspecific	
Busulfan	**Busulfan**	Cross-link DNA	Nonspecific	**Pulmonary fibrosis**, hyperpigmentation

TABLE 9-3	Antimetabolites			
DRUG CLASS	**DRUGS**	**MECHANISM OF ACTION**	**HARDCORE CELL-CYCLE PHASE**	**MAJOR SIDE EFFECTS**
Folate antagonists	**Methotrexate**	Inhibits dihydrofolate reductase	S phase	Myelosuppression, **hepatotoxicity**
Purine analogs	**6-mercaptopurine (6MP)**, *6-thioguanine*	Functionally incorporated into DNA/RNA		Neutropenia, rash
Pyrimidine analogs	**Fluorouracil (5-FU)**, *capecitabine*	Functionally incorporated into DNA/RNA		Hyperpigmentation, myelosuppression, and **neurotoxicity**
Pyrimidine antagonists	*Cytarabine arabinoside (Ara-C)*	Incorporated into DNA/RNA, terminate chain elongation	S phase	Myelosuppression, **granulocytopenia**

TABLE 9-4   Antibiotics

Drug Class	Drugs	Mechanism of Action	Hardcore Cell-Cycle Phase	Major Side Effects
Antibiotics	*Bleomycin*	Forms a ferrous iron-oxygen drug that complex/cleaves DNA	G2 phase	**Pulmonary fibrosis,** pneumonitis, Raynaud's phenomenon
	Dactinomycin	Intercalates with base pairs		Myelosuppression
	Actinomycin	Intercalates with base pairs		Myelosuppression
	Mitomycin C	Intercalating DNA/forms reactive oxidative radicals		Myelosuppression, **interstitial pneumonitis, nephrotoxicity**
	Doxorubicin (Adriamycin)	Intercalates between DNA base pairs, inhibits DNA topoisomerases I and II		**Cardiotoxicity**
	Daunorubicin	Intercalates between DNA base pairs, inhibits DNA topoisomerases I and II		**Cardiotoxicity**

TABLE 9-5   Microtubule Inhibitors

Drug Class	Drugs	Mechanism of Action	Hardcore Cell-Cycle Phase	Major Side Effects
Vinca alkaloids	*Vincristine*	Inhibits the polymerization of tubulin	M phase	Peripheral neuropathy
	Vinblastine	Inhibits the polymerization of tubulin	M phase	Myelosuppression, peripheral neuropathy
Taxols	*Paclitaxel*	Binds to tubulin and stabilizes microtubules	G2 and M phase	Myleosuppression, hepatic toxicity
	Docetaxel	Binds to tubulin and stabilizes microtubules	G2 and M phase	Myleosuppression, hepatic toxicity

TABLE 9-6   Topoisomerase Inhibitors

Drug Class	Drugs	Mechanism of Action	Hardcore Cell-Cycle Phase	Major Side Effects
Topoisomerase I inhibitors	*Topotecan*	Topoisomerase I inhibitor (blocks replication and transcription)	Late S and early G2 phase	Myelosuppression
Topoisomerase II inhibitors	*Etoposide*	Forms complex with topoisomerase II, blocks DNA replication/causes DNA strand breakage	Late S and early G2 phase	Myelosuppression, stomatitis

TABLE 9-7 Hormonal Agents

Drug Class	Drugs	Mechanism of Action	Hardcore Cell-Cycle Phase	Major Side Effects
Antiestrogens	*Tamoxifen*	Binds the estrogen receptor but induces no physiologic response		Menopausal symptoms, hepatotoxicity, **endometrial cancer**
	Raloxifene	Binds the estrogen receptor but induces no physiologic response		Menopausal symptoms, hepatotoxicity
Antiandrogens	*Flutamide*	Inhibits androgen uptake and binding		**Impotence**, gynecomastia
Aromatase inhibitors	*Anastrozole*	Inhibits the aromatase enzyme decreasing conversion of androgens to estrogen		Hot flashes, anorexia
	Letrozole	Inhibits the aromatase enzyme decreasing conversion of androgens to estrogen		Hot flashes, anorexia
LHRH agonists	*Leuprolide*	Increases LHRH release, suppressing FSH/LH		Weight gain, gynecomastia, depression
	Goserelin	Increases LHRH release, suppressing FSH/LH		Weight gain, gynecomastia, depression

TABLE 9-8 Monoclonal Antibodies

Drug Class	Drugs	Mechanism of Action	Hardcore Cell-Cycle Phase	Major Side Effects
Monoclonal Antibodies	*Rituximab*	Antibody directed at the CD20 surface antigen expressed on B-lymphocytes		**Hypersensitivity**, leukopenia, thrombocytopenia
	Imiximab	Antibody directed at the CD20 surface antigen expressed on B-lymphocytes		**Hypersensitivity**, leukopenia, thrombocytopenia

TABLE 9-9 Immunosuppressants

Drug Class	Drugs	Mechanism of Action	Major Side Effects
Nonselective immunosuppressants	*Azathioprine*	6-MP antagonizes purine metabolism, inhibiting the synthesis of DNA, RNA, and proteins	Bone marrow depression, hepatotoxicity
	Mycophenolate	Blocks the de novo formation of guanosine phosphate (GMP)	Leukopenia, sepsis, lymphoma
Selective immunosuppressants	*Cyclosporine*	Diffuses into T cells and forms a cyclosporin-cyclophillin complex that binds calcineurin and blocks cytokine release	Nephrotoxicity, hepatotoxicity, gingival hyperplasia
	Tacrolimus (FK506)	Diffuses into T cells and binds FK binding protein (FKBP) resulting in inhibition of cytokine synthesis	Nephrotoxicity, neurotoxicity
Antibodies	*Muromonab-CD3 (OKT3)*	Antibody directed against the CD3 antigen of human T cells	Anaphylaxis, seizures, encephalopathy

CHAPTER 10

Antimicrobials

A solid understanding of the fundamentals of antibiotic pharmacology is exceedingly important, as these concepts are more and more highly tested on the Step 1 exam. You should be familiar with the following:

- Class that each antibiotic belongs to
- Key enzyme(s) inhibited by the antimicrobial agent/class
- Mechanism of action, side effects, mechanisms of bacterial resistance, and major microbes affected by each antibiotic class
- Safe drugs for children
- Alternative drugs for patients allergic to the antibiotic of choice

The most hardcore antimicrobial concepts tested on Step 1 are mechanism of action, side effects, and resistance mechanisms, and there is less emphasis on indications and usage.

CELL WALL SYNTHESIS INHIBITORS

Natural penicillins: *Penicillin G, penicillin G benzanthine, penicillin G procaine, penicillin V*

β-lactamase-resistant penicillins: *Methicillin, nafcillin, oxacillin, dicloxacillin, cloxacillin*

Extended-coverage penicillins: *Amoxicillin, ampicillin*

Antipseudomonal penicillins: *Carbenicillin, piperacillin, ticarcillin*

β-lactamase inhibitors: *Clavulanic acid, sulbactam, tazobactam*

Antipseudomonal penicillins in combination with a β-lactamase inhibitor:
Piperacillin/tazobactam, ticarcillin/clavulanic acid

Extended-coverage penicillin in combination with a β-lactamase inhibitor:
Amoxicillin/clavulanic acid, ampicillin/sulbactam

Carbapenems: *Imipenem, meropenem, ertapenem*

Monobactam: *Aztreonam*

Cephalosporins: *First, second, third, fourth generations*

Vancomycin

General Characteristics of Cell Wall Synthesis Inhibitors (Except Vancomycin)

Mechanism of Action

- These compounds block the final step in bacterial cell wall synthesis by binding to and inhibiting **transpeptidase enzymes**. These enzymes are responsible for cross-linking of the peptidoglycan subunits of the bacterial cell wall.
- These compounds also activate bacterial enzymes called *endogenous autolysins* that are normally involved in the degradation and remodeling of the bacterial cell wall. Because transpeptidases are also inhibited, the cell wall is enzymatically degraded without being reconstructed.
- Bactericidal vs. bacteriostatic:
  - **Bactericidal**: The antibiotic *kills* the bacteria with the host immune system not required for bacterial killing.
  - **Bacteriostatic**: The antibiotic *stops* the growth of the bacteria, allowing the host immune system to fight bacteria more efficiently.

Side Effects—Key side effects of cell wall inhibitors include **allergic reaction** and rash. Additionally, if the administered antibiotic kills the normal colonic flora, *Clostridium difficile* overgrowth can occur, resulting in a superinfection and pseudomembranous enterocolitis

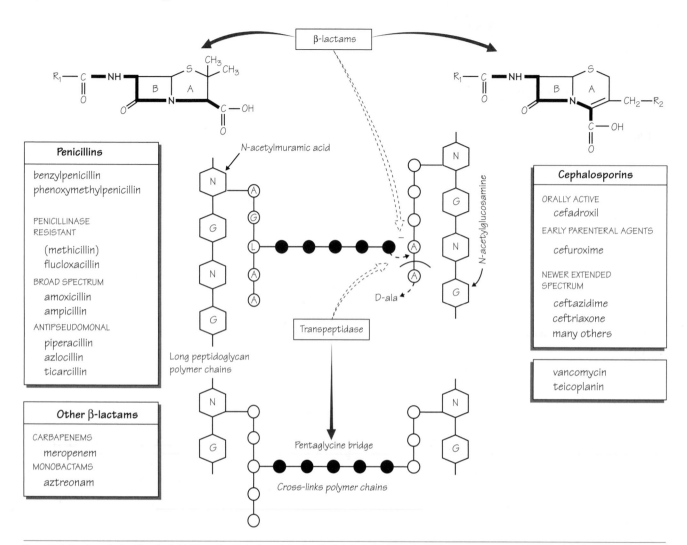

Figure 10-1 Overview of cell wall synthesis inhibitors. (Reprinted with permission from Neal MJ. Medical Pharmacology at a Glance. 4th ed. Oxford: Blackwell Publishing, 2002:82.)

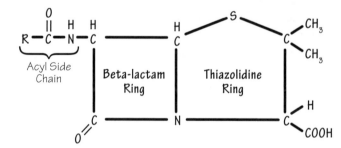

Figure 10-2 General structure of *penicillins*.
The β-lactam ring is the active site of the molecule.

Mechanisms of Bacterial Resistance to β-Lactam Antibiotics

1. <u>β-Lactamase-mediated inactivation</u>: β-lactamases are enzymes, produced by the bacteria, that hydrolytically cleave the β-lactam ring of the penicillins, which renders the antibiotic inactive.

Figure 10-3 Site of action of β-lactamase.

2. <u>Diminished permeability of the cell wall or outer membrane</u>: This prevents cell wall inhibitors from reaching the cell wall.

3. <u>Increased production of penicillin-binding proteins (PBPs)</u>: An increase in PBP production requires an increase in drug concentration to achieve the same therapeutic effect.

4. <u>Development of new PBPs</u>: Structurally unique PBPs have a decreased affinity for the β-lactam ring.

Natural Penicillins

 Penicillin G (IV, IM forms), penicillin V (oral form only)

These drugs are found in nature.

 Hardcore Bug Targets: **Gram (+) cocci, rods; gram (–) cocci; spirochetes**

Indications and Usage—Group A (*pyogenes*) and B (*agalactiae*) streptococci, *Streptococcus pneumoniae* (resistant strains are on the increase), *Peptostreptococcus*, syphilis (*Treponema pallidum*), *Neisseria meningitidis*, *Clostridium* spp.

- *Benzathine penicillin* G (IM form) is indicated for syphilis and streptococcal prophylaxis in patients with history of rheumatic fever (these are infections that require low levels of sustained antibiotic).
- *Penicillin V* is primarily used to treat mild infections of the throat, respiratory tract, or soft tissue.

Side Effects

- Allergic: Rash, urticaria, pruritus, bronchoconstriction, anaphylaxis, and erythema multiforme
- Gastrointestinal: Diarrhea, nausea, and vomiting
- Hematologic: Hemolytic anemia, neutropenia
- Neurologic: Potential muscle irritability and seizures in patients with renal failure

β-Lactamase-Resistant Penicillins

 Methicillin, nafcillin, oxacillin, dicloxacillin, cloxacillin

Resistant to degradation by β-lactamase.

 Hardcore Bug Targets: **Gram (+) cocci**

Indications and Usage—β-lactamase-producing *Staphylococcus* spp., primarily *Staphylococcus aureus*. Efficacious for penicillin-sensitive *S. pneumoniae* and group A streptococcus

Side Effects—Similar to penicillins; additionally, interstitial nephritis, liver toxicity, and thrombophlebitis

Extended-Coverage Penicillins

 Amoxicillin, ampicillin

Extended activity against the gram (–) bacilli.

 Hardcore Bug Targets: **Same as natural penicillin, with greater activity against gram (–) bacilli**

Indications and Usage—*S. pneumoniae*, group A streptococcus, and *N. meningitidis*. Also used for enterics: *Escherichia coli*, *Listeria*, *Proteus*, *Enterococcus*, *Salmonella*, and *Shigella*

- Extended-coverage penicillins are primarily used for the treatment of infections of the respiratory tract (sinusitis and bronchitis), ear, and genitourinary tract.

Side Effects—Similar to other penicillins; rashes and diarrhea are more common with *ampicillin* and *amoxicillin* than with any other *penicillins*.

Antipseudomonal Penicillins

 Carbenicillin, piperacillin, ticarcillin

Improved efficacy against gram (–) bacteria, but diminished efficacy against gram (+) bacteria.

 Hardcore Bug Targets—**Gram (–) rods, anaerobes**

Indications and Usage—*Pseudomonas*, *Proteus*, *Bacteroides*

Side Effects—Similar to other penicillins; additionally:

- *Piperacillin* and *ticarcillin* can cause platelet dysfunction.
- *Ticarcillin* and *carbenicillin* can cause hypokalemic alkalosis and/or sodium overload.

HARDCORE

Natural penicillins are not used empirically for *N. gonorrhoeae* or *S. pneumoniae* because of the rise in resistance.

HARDCORE

Methicillin is no longer used in the U.S. because of the high incidence of interstitial nephritis.

HARDCORE

β-Lactamase-resistant penicillins are **not degraded by β-lactamases** because their β-lactam ring is protected by bulky side chains.

HARDCORE

Amoxicillin is used before dental procedures for patients at risk for bacterial endocarditis.

HARDCORE

Patients with **mononucleosis** who are given *amoxicillin* or *ampicillin* are more likely to develop a rash.

HARDCORE

Antipseudomonal penicillins are sensitive to β-lactamase, so they are typically given in combination with β-lactamase inhibitors.

β-Lactamase Inhibitors

> *Clavulanic acid, sulbactam, tazobactam*

These drugs are not antibacterial if used alone.

Indications and Usage—These agents are used in combination with *penicillins* to target penicillin-resistant bacteria due to production of β-lactamase.

Mechanism of Action

- Bind irreversibly to β-lactamase catalytic site, thereby preventing the degradation of β-lactam antibiotics
- Bind directly to PBP, thereby enhancing the antibacterial action of the antibiotic

Antipseudomonal Penicillins in Combination with a β-Lactamase Inhibitor

> *Piperacillin/tazobactam, ticarcillin/clavulanic acid*

Indications and Usage—*Pseudomonas, Proteus, Bacteroides* (same as the antipseudomonal *penicillins*). Also β-lactamase-producing bacteria: *S. aureus, Haemophilus influenzae, Moraxella catarrhalis, N. gonorrhoeae, Proteus, Klebsiella, Bacteroides, Enterococcus*

Extended-Coverage Penicillin in Combination with a β-Lactamase Inhibitor

> *Amoxicillin/clavulanic acid, ampicillin/sulbactam*

Indications and Usage—*S. pneumoniae*, group A strep, and *N. meningitidis*. Also used for enterics: *E. coli, Klebsiella, Listeria, Proteus, Enterococcus, Salmonella,* and *Shigella* (same as the extended-coverage penicillins). In addition, other β-lactamase-producing bacteria: *S. aureus, H. influenzae, M. catarrhalis, N. gonorrhoeae, Haemophilus ducreyi, Bacteroides,* and dog-bite organisms

Carbapenems

> *Imipenem, meropenem, ertapenem*

The "-*penem*" group differs from *penicillins* by a substitution of a carbon atom for a sulfur atom and the addition of a double bond to the β-lactam ring. Similar to the penicillins, carbapenems prevent the elongation and cross-linking of bacterial cell wall peptidoglycan by inhibiting bacterial peptidases and PBPs. Carbapenems are considered "hardcore" antibiotics because of their broad spectrum of antimicrobial activity and resistance to a broad range of β-lactamases present in gram (+), gram (−), and anaerobic bacteria.

Hardcore Bug Targets: **Broad spectrum; aerobic gram (+) and gram (−), and anaerobes**

Indications and Usage—Reserved for serious mixed polymicrobial infections in which aerobic gram (−) rods and anaerobes are all involved

Side Effects—Seizures with *imipenem*; *penicillin*-associated allergic reactions, GI disturbances, and skin rashes

Monobactam

> *Aztreonam*

Alternative to aminoglycosides (see aminoglycoside section below).

Hardcore Bug Targets: **Limited to aerobic gram (−) rods. No activity against gram (+) cocci or anaerobes**

Indications and Usage—Enterobacteriaceae (*E. coli, Klebsiella, Proteus*), *Serratia* spp., and *Pseudomonas*

Side Effects—Pain at the injection site, GI discomfort, hepatotoxicity, and rarely thrombocytopenia

Cephalosporins

> **First generation:** *Cefazolin, cephalexin*
> **Second generation:** *Cefuroxime, cefoxitin, cefotetan*
> **Third generation:** *Ceftriaxone, cefotaxime, ceftazidime, cefixime*
> **Fourth generation:** *Cefepime*

These agents are classified into four generations that coincide with their spectrum of activity against gram (−) organisms. In general, all are active against gram (+) cocci, but with a decrease in effectiveness from the first to the third generations. The exception to this rule is the fourth-generation cephalosporin *cefepime*, which has broad-spectrum antibiotic coverage and good activity against gram (+) bacteria. In contrast, antibiotic activity against gram (−) organisms increases in effectiveness from the first generation to fourth generation of cephalosporins.

With the exception of *ceftriaxone* (third generation), cephalosporins are eliminated via renal active tubular secretion and glomerular filtration. Due to the route of elimination, dosage adjustments are necessary in patients with renal insufficiency

Mechanism of Action—Same as the *penicillins*

Side Effects—Cephalosporins are generally well tolerated:

- Immunologic: Cross-allergic reactions occur in *10% to 15% of patients allergic to penicillin*. Symptoms include maculopapular rash, urticaria, fever, eosinophilia, and thrombophlebitis with IV administration.
- GI: Nausea, vomiting, and diarrhea; pseudomembranous colitis caused by C. *difficile* overgrowth
- Hematologic: Increased prothrombin time due to the inhibition of vitamin K-dependent clotting factor synthesis
- Other: *Cefotetan* (second generation) can cause a *disulfuram*-like reaction after ingestion of alcohol; patients may develop cholelithiasis (gallstones) with *ceftriaxone*

FIRST GENERATION

 Cefazolin, cephalexin

 Hardcore Bug Targets: High gram (+) coverage and limited gram (−) coverage

Indications and Usage—*Staphylococcus* spp., *Streptococcus* spp., Enterobacteriaceae

- *Proteus, E. coli, Klebsiella*: PEcK

SECOND GENERATION

 Cefuroxime, cefoxitin, cefotetan

Hardcore Bug Targets: Decreased gram (+) coverage and increased gram (−) coverage

Indications and Usage—*Staphylococcus* spp. (not as effective as first generation), *Streptococcus* spp., anaerobes including *Bacteroides*

- *H. influenzae, Neisseria* spp., *Proteus, E. coli, Klebsiella*: HiNPEcK

THIRD GENERATION

 Ceftriaxone, cefotaxime, ceftazidime, cefixime

Hardcore Bug Targets: Decreased gram (+) coverage and increased gram (−) coverage

Indications and Usage—*Staphylococcus* spp. (*not as effective as first generation*), *Streptococcus* spp., and *Pseudomonas* spp.

- *H. influenzae, Neisseria* spp., *Proteus, E. coli, Klebsiella*, Serratia: HiNPEcKS
- *Ceftriaxone* and *cefixime* are the drugs of choice for the treatment of gonorrhea (*Neisseria gonorrhoeae*)

FOURTH GENERATION

 Cefepime

Hardcore Bug Targets: Increased gram (+) coverage and increased gram (−) coverage

Indications and Usage—*Staphylococcus* spp., *Streptococcus* spp.

- *H. influenzae, Enterobacter, Neisseria* spp., Proteus, *Pseudomonas aeruginosa, E. coli, Citrobacter, Klebsiella, Serratia*: HiNPEcKS

Vancomycin

A glycopeptide antimicrobial.

Hardcore Bug Targets: Limited to aerobic and anaerobic gram (+) bacteria

Indications and Usage—*S. aureus*, methicillin-resistant *S. aureus* (MRSA), *Staphylococcus epidermidis*, methicillin-resistant *S. epidermidis* (MRSE), *S. pneumoniae*, penicillin-resistant *S. pneumoniae*, *C. difficile, Clostridium perfringens, Enterococcus, Listeria*

Mechanism of Action—Inhibition of peptidoglycan synthesis:

- *Vancomycin* binds to the bacterial *d-alanyl-d-alanine* portion of a pentapeptide involved in the peptidoglycan synthesis.

HARDCORE

The following organisms are **not susceptible** to *cephalosporins*:

- **MRSA**: Use vancomycin
- **Enterococci**: Use ampicillin
- **C. difficile**: Use metronidazole
- **Listeria**: Use ampicillin or penicillin
- Organisms causing atypical pneumonia, including **Legionella**, **Mycoplasma**, and **Chlamydia**

HARDCORE

The second-generation cephalosporins *cefoxitin* and *cefotetan* are the only cephalosporins **active against** *Bacteroides*.

HARDCORE

The third-generation cephalosporin *ceftazidime* and the fourth-generation cephalosporin *cefepime* are the only cephalosporins **effective against** *P. aeruginosa*.

HARDCORE

First-generation cephalosporins are used clinically for skin and soft tissue infections, as well as for prophylaxis of wound infections following surgery.

HARDCORE

Vancomycin is reserved for serious infections by MRSA, MRSE, or other β-lactam-sensitive strains in patients with β-lactam allergies.

HARDCORE

Vancomycin is the second choice for pseu' domembranous colitis (*C. difficile*). The dr' of choice is *metronidazole* taken orally.

- The *d-alanyl-d-alanine-vancomycin* complex prevents both peptidoglycan polymerase and transpeptidase reactions from occurring.

Enterococcus Resistance to Vancomycin—An alteration of the terminal amino acid of the pentapeptide results in resistance. Vancomycin-resistant enterococci (VRE) have three major phenotypes: *VanA, VanB, and VanC*

1. **VanA and VanB**:

   a. The most frequently encountered phenotypes. They possess the highest level of *vancomycin* resistance.

   b. Acquired through transmissible elements located on plasmids, and can also be inserted into chromosomes

   c. Encode an enzyme that produces *d-Ala-d-**Lactate** dipeptide*. Vancomycin is unable to bind this dipeptide.

2. **VanC**:

   a. Possess a lower level of *vancomycin* resistance than VanA or VanB

   b. Intrinsic to organisms

   c. Encode an enzyme that produces *d-Ala-d-**Serine** dipeptide*

S. aureus Resistance to Vancomycin—Vancomycin-intermediate *S. aureus* (VISA) and vancomycin-resistant *S. aureus* (VRSA) are resistant to *vancomycin*. Mechanisms by which resistance occurs have not been clearly defined; however, it has been shown that the genes responsible for enterococci resistance are not responsible for *S. aureus* resistance.

Side Effects—Thrombophlebitis, fever, chills, neutropenia, ototoxicity (especially in combination with an aminoglycoside)

PROTEIN SYNTHESIS INHIBITORS

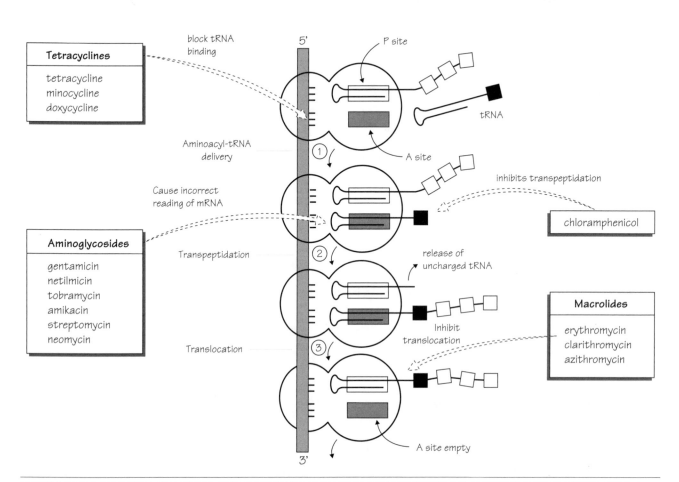

Figure 10-4 Overview of the protein synthesis inhibitors. Protein synthesis inhibitors act on various sites within the bacterial ribosomal assembly line for proteins, to prevent the synthesis of proteins. (Reprinted with permission from Neal MJ. Medical Pharmacology at a Glance. 4th ed. Oxford: Blackwell Publishing, 2002:84.)

Macrolides: *Erythromycin, clarithromycin, azithromycin*

Aminoglycosides: *Gentamicin, tobramycin, amikacin, streptomycin, spectinomycin*

Tetracyclines: *Tetracycline, doxycycline, minocycline, demeclocycline*

Chloramphenicol

Streptogramins

Oxazolidiones: *Linezolid*

Macrolides

Erythromycin, clarithromycin, azithromycin

The "-thromycins."

⊕ *Hardcore Bug Targets*: Gram (+), atypical, and minimal gram (−) coverage

Indications and Usage—*S. pneumoniae* and other streptococci and staphylococci. Also, atypical organisms including *Mycobacterium, Legionella, Mycoplasma,* and *Chlamydia* spp.

- *Clarithromycin* is used as part of triple therapy against peptic ulcer disease associated with *Helicobacter pylori* (with *amoxicillin* and *metronidazole*).
- *Clarithromycin* and *azithromycin* are effective against upper respiratory infection caused by *S. pneumoniae, H. influenza,* or *M. catarrhalis.*

Mechanism of Action—Inhibition of RNA-dependent protein synthesis by reversibly binding to the **50S ribosomal subunit** of the 70S bacterial ribosome, resulting in dissociation of tRNA from the ribosome

Side Effects—GI disturbances including nausea, vomiting, diarrhea, and abdominal cramps are more common with *erythromycin*, but can occur with all macrolides. All macrolides can cause ventricular tachycardia, prolongation of the QT interval, and torsades de pointes.

Aminoglycosides

Gentamicin, tobramycin, amikacin, streptomycin, spectinomycin

⊕ *Hardcore Bug Targets*: Gram (−) enteric bacteria and *Pseudomonas*

Indications and Usage—*P. aeruginosa,* Enterobacteriaceae (*E. coli, Klebsiella, Proteus, Enterobacter*)

- Aminoglycosides are synergistic with β-lactam antibiotics for gram (−) infections.
- Streptomycin is used exclusively against tularemia (caused by *Francisella tularensis*), plague (*Yersinia pestis*), in combination with tetracycline for brucellosis (*Brucella abortus*), and in combination with other antituberculosis drugs (see Chapter 11).
- Spectinomycin is useful only for *N. gonorrhoeae* infections.

Mechanism of Action—Bind irreversibly to the **30S subunit of the bacterial ribosome**, interfering with either the formation of an initiation complex or with translation of the genetic code, ultimately inhibiting bacterial protein synthesis

HARDCORE

Protein synthesis inhibitors (**except the aminoglycosides**) are considered **bacteriostatic**, i.e., they do not kill the bacteria themselves, but prevent further bacterial growth, allowing the host's immune system to eliminate invading bugs.

HARDCORE

Human cells have 80S ribosomes and are not affected by macrolides.

HARDCORE

Erythromycin strongly **inhibits CYP450** and can result in increased levels of medications metabolized by CYP450. *Clarithromycin* also inhibits CYP450, but to a lesser extent.

HARDCORE

Amikacin is mainly used for organisms resistant to other aminoglycosides, because of its resistance to inactivating enzymes.

HARDCORE

Aminoglycosides are unique, because their antibacterial killing activity can continue even after serum drug concentrations decline below the minimum inhibitory concentration (MIC); this is known as the **post-antibiotic effect**.

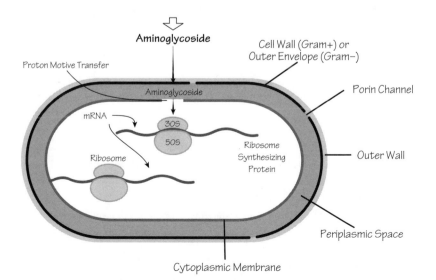

Figure 10-5 Aminoglycoside mechanism of action.

HARDCORE

High aminoglycoside doses can produce neuromuscular blockade and paralysis. This paralysis can be reversed in the early stages by a calcium infusion or by neostigmine.

HARDCORE

Demeclocycline is used only to treat patients with syndrome of inappropriate antidiuretic hormone (SIADH).

HARDCORE

Absorption of the *tetracyclines* may be impaired by multivalent cations (including Ca^{2+}, Mg^{2+}, Fe^{2+}, Al^{3+}); therefore, they should not be taken with food, dairy products, multivitamins, or antacids.

HARDCORE

Tetracyclines are associated with decreased bone growth if given during pregnancy, and **decreased bone growth and teeth discoloration if given to children** younger than 8 years old.

HARDCORE

Clindamycin may be used for staphylococcal infections and before dental procedures as part of endocarditis prophylaxis in patients allergic to *penicillin.*

HARDCORE

On board exams (and on the wards), *clindamycin* use is commonly associated with **C. difficile** *overgrowth* (due to the antibiotic killing of natural colonic flora), which can result in the development of pseudo-membranous colitis.

HARDCORE

Chloramphenicol should be used only for serious infections, because of its serious side effects.

HARDCORE

In addition to the bacterial 50S ribosomal subunit, mammalian mitochondrial ribosomal RNA (70S) is also capable of binding *chloramphenicol.* This can result in dose-related bone marrow suppression.

Mechanisms of Bacterial Resistance to Aminoglycosides

- Inactivation by enzyme-mediated covalent modification; a phosphate, adenyl, or acetyl group is transferred to the aminoglycoside, resulting in decreased affinity for the bacterial ribosome
- Ribosomal mutation can result in decreased drug affinity for the 30S ribosomal subunit
- Decreased bacterial drug uptake

Side Effects—Ototoxicity (irreversible) and nephrotoxicity (reversible)

Tetracyclines

 Tetracycline, doxycycline, minocycline, demeclocycline

Hardcore Bug Targets: **Broad spectrum, including gram (+), gram (−), anaerobes, atypical bacteria, and protozoan parasites**

Indications and Usage—Nongonococcal urethritis (i.e., *Chlamydia trachomatis, Ureaplasma urealyticum*), atypical pneumonia (e.g., *Chlamydia pneumoniae, Legionella* spp., *Mycoplasma* spp.), community-acquired pneumonia (e.g., *S. pneumoniae, H. influenzae*), others (e.g., *Y. pestis, Bartonella* spp., *Borrelia burgdorferi*)

Mechanism of Action—Inhibits protein synthesis by **binding to the bacterial 30S and 50S ribosomal subunits**

Side Effects—Nausea, vomiting, and diarrhea are most common; photosensitivity may also occur with sun exposure.

Clindamycin

Hardcore Bug Targets: **Aerobic gram (+) cocci, anaerobes**

Indications and Usage—Mouth anaerobes (peptococcus, peptostreptococcus, and/or *Fusobacterium* spp.), *Propionibacterium acnes* (associated with acne), *Clostridium* spp., *Bacteroides, S. aureus* (except MRSA), *Streptococcus* spp.

Mechanism of Action—Inhibits protein synthesis by reversibly **binding to the bacterial 50S ribosomal subunit**

Side Effects—Severe diarrhea, nausea, and vomiting

Chloramphenicol

Hardcore Bug Targets: **Broad-spectrum antibiotic**

Indications and Usage—Meningitis pathogens (*S. pneumoniae, H. influenzae, N. meningitidis*), anaerobes (*Bacteroides*), Enterococcus, *Salmonella typhi, Rickettsia* spp.

Mechanism of Action—Inhibits protein synthesis by **binding to the bacterial 50S ribosomal subunit**

Side Effects—Dose-related bone marrow suppression, idiosyncratic aplastic anemia, *gray baby syndrome*

Streptogramins

 Quinupristin-dalfopristin

This group is composed of a pair of synergistic constituents, quinupristin, and dalfopristin.

Hardcore Bug Targets—**Gram (+), atypical, and minimal gram (−) coverage**

Indications and Usage—MRSA, *VRE*, macrolide- or penicillin-resistant pneumococci, and the treatment of gram (+) cocci infections in patients not able to tolerate a more conventional agent

Mechanism of Action—Inhibits protein synthesis by **binding to the bacterial 50S ribosomal subunit**, thereby preventing the incorporation of the aminoacyl tRNA into the cellular ribosome and the translation of mRNA

Side Effects

- Moderate and transient elevation of liver enzymes at high doses
- Allergic reaction that leads to itching, burning, and erythema of the front of the neck and upper torso
- Potent inhibitor of cytochrome P-450
- QT interval prolongation when administered with drugs metabolized by 3A4

Oxazolidinone

 Linezolid

This class is considered an alternative for the treatment of resistant gram (+) infections.

Hardcore Bug Targets: Gram (+) bacteria, anaerobes

Indications and Usage—*Staphylococcus* spp., *Streptococcus* spp., *Enterococcus* spp., and *Listeria monocytogenes*

- Used for resistant bacteria: MRSA, VISA, penicillin-resistant *S. pneumoniae*, and VRE
- Moderately active against anaerobes (*Clostridium* spp., *Peptococcus* spp., *Bacteroides fragilis*, and *Fusobacterium* spp.)

Mechanism of Action—Protein synthesis inhibition via binding to **bacterial 70S ribosome initiation complex**

Side Effects—Nausea, diarrhea, headaches. In addition, thrombocytopenia, which is completely reversible on discontinuation of the drug

HARDCORE

No cross-resistance exists between the *oxazolidinones* and other protein synthesis inhibitors, because this class acts on a different stage of protein synthesis (during the initiation complex formation).

HARDCORE

Linezolid is a weak monoamine oxidase (MAO) inhibitor, so patients using it should avoid tyramine-rich foods and drugs with serotonergic and/or adrenergic effects (see Chapter 2).

DNA SYNTHESIS INHIBITORS

 First generation: *Nalidixic acid (not used clinically or tested on Step 1)*

Second generation: *Norfloxacin, ofloxacin, ciprofloxacin*

Third generation: *Levofloxacin, gatifloxacin, moxifloxacin*

Fourth generation: *Trovafloxacin*

Quinolones (First Generation Only) and Fluoroquinolones (Second Through Fourth Generations)

These agents are classified into four generations according to their spectrum of activity. In general, all four generations are active against gram (–) bacteria and intestinal pathogens, but have increasing activity against gram (+) and atypical bacteria from the first generation to the fourth generation. In addition, the fourth generation *fluoroquinolones* are active against anaerobes and thus are considered broad-spectrum antibiotics.

General Characteristics of the Fluoroquinolones

Mechanism of Action—Inhibit **topoisomerase type II** (also known as DNA gyrase) and **topoisomerase type IV**, causing termination of DNA replication

Side Effects

- GI: Upset stomach, fatal liver toxicity (associated only with trovafloxacin)
- Allergic: Rash, urticaria, photosensitivity
- Cardiac: QT prolongation
- Musculoskeletal: Chondrocyte toxicity causing **impaired cartilage development**. Therefore should not be given to pregnant women, breast feeding women, or children

Second Generation

 Norfloxacin, ofloxacin, ciprofloxacin

 Hardcore Bug Targets: Gram (–), gram (+), genitourinary (GU) bugs

Indications and Usage—Enterobacteriaceae (*E. coli, Klebsiella, Proteus, Enterobacter*), *P. aeruginosa*, GU bugs (*Neisseria, C. trachomatis, Mycoplasma hominis*), *Bartonella, Legionella*, moderate staphylococcal activity

Third Generation

 Levofloxacin, gatifloxacin, moxifloxacin

The "respiratory" quinolones.

 Hardcore Bug Targets: Gram (–), gram (+), GU pathogens (especially the respiratory bugs and atypicals)

Indications and Usage—Same coverage as second generation DNA synthesis inhibitors, but with the addition of coverage against *S. pneumoniae* and atypical bacteria (*C. pneumoniae, Mycoplasma pneumoniae, H. influenzae, M. catarrhalis*, and *Mycobacterium* spp.)

Fourth Generation

 Trovafloxacin

 Hardcore Bug Targets: Gram (–), gram (+), respiratory pathogens, GU pathogens, atypicals, anaerobes

HARDCORE

Topoisomerases are bacterial enzymes that help maintain DNA in an appropriate state of supercoiling.

- **Topoisomerase II** functions in negative supercoiling and elimination of supercoils at the replication fork.
- **Topoisomerase IV** functions in the separation of daughter DNA molecules after replication is complete.

HARDCORE

Ciprofloxacin is the most active quinolone against *Pseudomonas*.

HARDCORE

Because of the risk of fatal hepatotoxicity, *trovafloxacin* is used only for life-threatening infections in hospitalized patients for whom the benefits of the drug outweigh the risks.

HARDCORE

The combination of *TMP* and *SMX* is synergistic.

HARDCORE

Avoid using sulfa drugs in patients with **glucose 6-phosphate dehydrogenase (G6PD) deficiency**, because they can produce hemolytic anemia.

HARDCORE

Nitrofurantoin is metabolized and excreted in the kidneys, and may cause a brown discoloration of the urine.

Indications and Usage—Same spectrum as above with the addition of anaerobes

Sulfonamides

Trimethoprim-sulfamethoxazole (TMP-SMX), sulfadiazine, sulfisoxazole

Hardcore Bug Targets: **Enteric gram (−), limited gram (+)**

Indications and Usage—*S. aureus*; *S. pneumoniae*; GU bugs (*E. coli, Klebsiella, Enterobacter, Proteus, Serratia*); others (*Nocardia, Actinomyces, Listeria, Toxoplasma, Plasmodium, Pneumocystis carinii*, which causes *P. carinii* pneumonia [PCP])

Mechanism of Action—Inhibition of bacterial DNA synthesis via:

1. Trimethoprim (TMP): Inhibits **dihydrofolate reductase**, the enzyme responsible for the conversion of dihydrofolate to tetrahydrofolate
2. Sulfamethoxazole (SMX), sulfadiazine, and sulfisoxazole: Inhibit **dihydropteroate synthetase**, the enzyme responsible for the conversion of PABA to folic acid

Side Effects

- Allergic: Rash, photosensitivity, **Stevens-Johnson syndrome**
- GI: Nausea, vomiting, hepatotoxicity (rare)
- Hematologic: Anemia, leukopenia

Others

Nitrofurantoin

Indications and Usage—**Gram (+) and gram (−) aerobes**. For prophylaxis and treatment of urinary tract infections caused by *E. coli, Klebsiella*, enterococci, *S. aureus*. Not useful in UTIs caused by *Proteus* or *Pseudomonas*

Mechanism of Action—Nitrofurantoin is reduced by bacterial enzymes to **reactive intermediates**, which inactivate or alter bacterial ribosomal proteins and other macromolecules, resulting in inhibition of protein synthesis, energy metabolism, DNA and RNA synthesis, and cell wall synthesis

Side Effects

- GI: Anorexia, nausea, stomach upset, and vomiting are the most common
- Allergic: Allergic pulmonary infiltrates/pneumonitis, lupus-like syndrome
- Hematologic: Hemolytic anemia in patients with G6PD deficiency

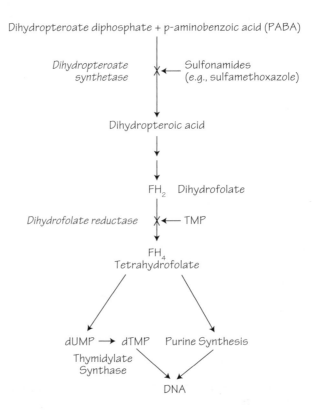

Figure 10-6 Mechanism of action of trimethoprim-sulfamethoxazole.

HARDCORE REVIEW – ANTIMICROBIAL PHARMACOLOGY

TABLE 10-1	Drugs Effective Against "Special" Bacteria			
BACTERIA	**GRAM STAIN**	**MORPHOLOGY**	**HARDCORE DRUGS OF CHOICE**	**ALTERNATIVES**
MRSA	+	Diplococci in pairs	*Vancomycin*	*Cinezolid, quinupristin/dalfopristin*
VRE	+	Cocci in chains	*Linezolid*	*Quinupristin/dalfopristin*
Pseudomonas	–	Rods	*Cefipime, ceftazidime, piperacillin/tazobactam, ticarcillin/clavulanic acid*	*Aminoglycosides, carbapenems*
N. gonorrhoeae	–	Intracellular diplococci	*Ceftriaxone, cefixime*	*Penicillin G, spectinomycin*
N. meningitidis	–	Intracellular diplococci	*Penicillin G*	*Third-generation cephalosporin, (rifampin is given as prophylactic agent to close contacts)*
T. pallidum (syphilis)	–	Spirochete	*Penicillin G*	*Doxycycline, azithromycin*
Bacteroides	–	Bacillus encapsulated anaerobes	*Clindamycin, metronidazole* (Chapter 11)	*Imipenem, meropenem, antipseudomonal penicillins*

TABLE 10-2	The Cell Wall Synthesis Inhibitors			
DRUG CLASS	**DRUGS**	**HARDCORE BUG TARGETS**	**MECHANISM OF ACTION**	**MAJOR SIDE EFFECTS**
Natural penicillins	*Penicillin G, penicillin V*	• Gram (+) cocci/rods • Gram (–) cocci • Spirochetes	Inhibition of transpeptidases	Anaphylaxis, erythema multiforme, hemolytic anemia
β-lactamase-resistant penicillins	*Methicillin, nafcillin, oxacillin, dicloxacillin, cloxacillin*	• Gram (+) cocci	Inhibition of transpeptidases	Liver toxicity, thrombophlebitis, interstitial nephritis
Extended-coverage penicillins	*Amoxicillin, ampicillin*	• Gram (+) cocci/rods • Gram (–) cocci • Spirochetes • *Greater activity against gram (–) bacilli*	Inhibition of transpeptidases	Rashes and diarrhea
Antipseudomonal penicillins	*Carbenicillin, ticarcillin, piperacillin*	• Gram (–) rods • Anaerobes	Inhibition of transpeptidases	Hypokalemic alkalosis, platelet dysfunction
Penicillin combined with a β-lactamase inhibitor	*Ampicillin/sulbactam, amoxicillin/clavulanic acid, piperacillin/tazobactam*	• Gram (+)	Inhibition of transpeptidases	Same as above for each specific component of the combination. β-lactamase inhibitors are not associated with significant side effects
Carbapenems	*Imipenem-cilastatin, meropenem, ertapenem*	**Broad spectrum** • Aerobes • Gram (+) • Gram (–) • Anaerobes	Inhibition of transpeptidases	*Imipenem* is nephrotoxic if not given with *cilastatin*; seizures
Monobactams	*Aztreonam*	• Aerobic gram (–) rods	Inhibition of transpeptidases	Pain at injection site, thrombocytopenia
Vancomycin	*Vancomycin*	• Aerobic gram (+) • Anaerobic gram (+)	Inhibition of peptidoglycan synthesis	Thrombophlebitis, neutropenia, red man syndrome
Cephalosporins			Inhibition of transpeptidases	Allergic reactions/rash and pseudomembranous colitis
1st generation	*Cefazolin, cephalexin*	• High gram (+) • Limited gram (–)		
2nd generation	*Cefuroxime, cefoxitin, cefotetan*	• Decreased gram (+) • Increased gram (–)		*Disulfuram*-like reaction with *cefotetan*
3rd generation	*Ceftriaxone, cefotaxime, ceftazidime*	• Increasingly limited gram (+) • Increased gram (–)		Cholelithiasis with *ceftriaxone*
4th generation	*Cefepime*	• Increased gram (+) • Increased gram (–)		

TABLE 10-3 Protein Synthesis Inhibitors

Drug Class	Drugs	Hardcore Bug Targets	Mechanism of Action	Major Side Effects
Macrolides	*Erythromycin, azithromycin, clarithromycin*	• Gram (+) • Atypicals • Minimal gram (−)	Inhibition of **50S** ribosomal subunit	Diarrhea, prolongation of the QT interval → torsades de pointes, *erythromycin* strongly inhibits CYP-450
Aminoglycosides	*Spectinomycin gentamicin, tobramycin, amikacin, streptomycin,*	• Gram (−) • Enteric bacteria *Pseudomonas*	Inhibition of **30S** ribosomal subunit	Ototoxicity (irreversible), nephrotoxicity
Tetracyclines	*Tetracycline, doxycycline, minocycline, demeclocycline*	*Broad spectrum* • Gram (+) • Gram (−) • Anaerobes • Atypical bacteria • Protozoan parasites	Inhibition of both **30S** and **50S** ribosomal subunits	Photosensitivity, decreased bone growth, discoloration of teeth
Clindamycin	*Clindamycin*	• Aerobic gram (+) cocci • Anaerobes	Inhibition of **50S** ribosomal subunit	Severe diarrhea, pseudomembranous colitis
Chloramphenicol	*Chloramphenicol*	*Broad spectrum*	Inhibition of **50S** ribosomal subunit	Dose-related bone marrow suppression, aplastic anemia, **gray baby syndrome**
Streptogramins	*Quinupristin-dalfopristin*	• Gram (+) • Atypicals • Minimal gram (−)	Inhibition of **50S** ribosomal subunit	Pain and erythema at injection site, liver enzyme elevation, prolongation of QT interval
Oxazolidinones	*Linezolid*	• Gram (+) • Anaerobes	Inhibition of **70S** ribosomal *initiation-complex*	Reversible thrombocytopenia, serotonin-like syndrome

TABLE 10-4 DNA Synthesis Inhibitors

Drug Class	Drugs	Hardcore Bug Targets	Mechanism of Action	Major Side Effects
Fluoroquinolones			Inhibition of topoisomerase II (DNA gyrase) and topoisomerase IV	Photosensitivity, QT prolongation → torsades de pointes, impaired cartilage development (*therefore not to be used during pregnancy or for children*)
Second generation	*Norfloxacin, ofloxacin, ciprofloxacin*	• Gram (−) • Gram (+) • Genitourinary		
Third generation	*Levofloxacin, gatifloxacin, moxifloxacin*	• Gram (−) • Gram (+) genitourinary • Respiratory bugs • Typicals		
Fourth generation	*Trovafloxacin*	• Gram (−) • Gram (+) • Respiratory • Genitourinary • Atypicals • Anaerobes		Fatal liver toxicity
Sulfonamides	*Trimethoprim-sulfamethoxazole (TMP-SMX), sulfadiazine, sulfisoxazole*	• Enteric gram (−) • Limited gram (+)	*Trimethoprim* → Inhibition of dihydrofolate reductase *Sulfa drugs* → Inhibition of dihydropteroate synthetase	Photosensitivity, Stevens-Johnson syndrome, hemolytic anemia in patients with G6PD deficiency, leukopenia

CHAPTER 11

Antifungal, Antimycobacterial, Antiviral, and Antiparasitic Pharmacology

Drugs in this chapter are among the least tested (but the most dense to study) on the USMLE Step 1. Keeping this in mind, you should focus on the mechanisms of important drugs and general drug classes, the key enzymes inhibited, and distinguishing or unique side effects.

ANTIFUNGALS

Subcutaneous and systemic antifungals: *Amphotericin B, capsofungin, flucytosine, terbinafine*

Topical antifungals: *Nystatin, griseofulvin*

Imidazoles

    Systemic imidazoles: *Fluconazole, itraconazole, ketoconazole, voriconazole*

    Topical imidazoles: *Clotrimazole, miconazole, ketoconazole*

Fungi are eukaryotic organisms with rigid cell walls that contain **chitin and glucan**, and cell membranes that contain **ergosterol**, a derivative of cholesterol. These characteristics account for the general fungal resistance to antibiotic agents and are targets for antifungal drugs. Clinically, fungal infections are typically superficial and involve the skin or mucous membranes, but can also be quite serious, causing systemic complications that necessitate urgent intervention.

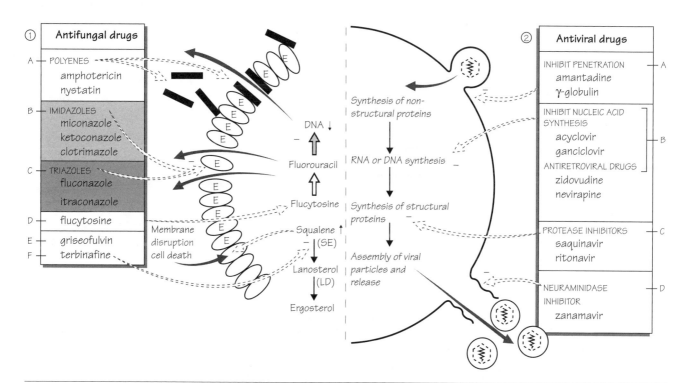

Figure 11-1 Overview of antifungal and antiviral drugs. (1) Antifungals act through several different mechanisms to disrupt both fungal ergosterol synthesis and function, and fungal DNA synthesis and replication: **polyenes (a)** form pores in ergosterol; **imidazoles (b)** and **triazoles (c)** inhibit ergosterol synthesis; **flucytosine (d)** inhibits DNA synthesis; **griseofulvin (e)** inhibits fungal microtubule function; and **terbinafine (f)** inhibits squalene epoxide, resulting in toxic levels of squalene within the fungal cell. **(2) Antivirals** act to inhibit viral penetration of the host cell **(a)**; viral replication within the host cell **(b and c)**; and the assembly and release of viral particles **(d)**. (Reprinted with permission from Neal MJ. Medical Pharmacology at a Glance. 4th ed. Oxford: Blackwell Publishing, 2002:86.)

Subcutaneous and Systemic Antifungals

 Amphotericin B, capsofungin, flucytosine, terbinafine

AMPHOTERICIN B

Indications and Usage—Serious fungal infections caused by *Candida*, *Cryptococcus*, *Histoplasmosis*, *Blastomyces*, *Coccidioides*, *Aspergillus*, and *Mucor*; amphotericin B is the most active antifungal drug for all systemic mycoses

Mechanism of Action—Binds to **ergosterol** and forms **membrane pores** that alter fungal cell membrane permeability and cause fungal cell lysis

Side Effects—*Amphotericin* is often referred to as "**amphoterrible**" due to its multiple side effects:

- **Acute infusion related reaction**: **Chills**, hypotension, and vomiting are common after IV infusion
- **Renal**: **Nephrotoxicity**
- **Hypotension and hypokalemia**
- **Thrombophlebitis**: Use heparin with infusion to avoid this complication
- **Anemia**: Secondary to reversible suppression of erythrocyte production

CASPOFUNGIN

Indications and Usage—Infections caused by *Candida* or *Aspergillus*

Mechanism of Action—Blocks cell wall synthesis by **inhibiting β-1,3 glucan synthase** and preventing the formation of β-glucan, a key cell wall component

Side Effects—Histamine-mediated symptoms including rash, facial swelling, pruritus, or bronchospasm

FLUCYTOSINE

Indications and Usage—Subcutaneous chromomycosis and in conjunction with *amphotericin B* for systemic deep fungal infections caused by *Candida, Cryptococcus, or Aspergillus*

Mechanism of Action—Acts inside fungal cells as a pyrimidine antimetabolite. Flucytosine is converted to **5-fluorouracil**, which is subsequently converted to 5-fluorodeoxyuridine monophosphate (**5-FdUMP**). **5-FdUMP inhibits thymidylate synthase**, an enzyme necessary for the DNA synthesis.

Side Effects—Elevated liver enzymes, neutropenia, and thrombocytopenia due to **bone marrow suppression**

- *Flu<u>cytosin</u>e* is <u>Cyto</u>logically <u>Sin</u>-ful, causing neutropenia and thrombocytopenia

TERBINAFINE

Indications and Usage—Nail infections, specifically for onychomycosis; dermatophytes

Mechanism of Action—**Blocks ergosterol synthesis** by inhibiting squalene epoxidase, altering permeability, ultimately resulting in cell lysis

Side Effects—GI distress, **loss of sense of taste**

Topical Antifungals

 Nystatin, griseofulvin

NYSTATIN

Indications and Usage—Cutaneous or mucocutaneous (oral/vaginal) *Candidiasis*

Mechanism of Action—**Binds to ergosterol** and **disrupts** fungal cell membranes, altering permeability, ultimately resulting in cell lysis

Side Effects—Rare when used topically

GRISEOFULVIN

Indications and Usage—Dermatophyte infections (*Microsporum, Epidermophyton, Trichophyton*), and also for infections involving **tinea capitis**

Mechanism of Action—**Inhibits fungal microtubule function**

Side Effects—Pancytopenia, renal toxicity

Imidazoles

 Systemic: *Fluconazole, itraconazole, ketoconazole, voriconazole*
Topical: *Clotrimazole, miconazole, ketoconazole*

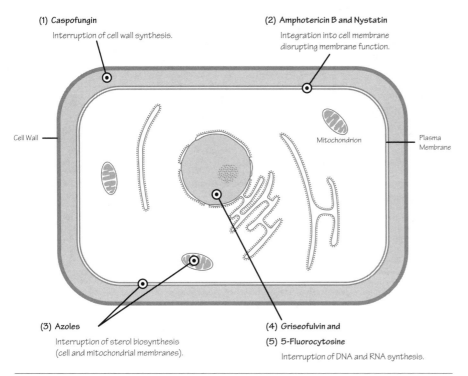

(1) Caspofungin
Interruption of cell wall synthesis.

(2) Amphotericin B and Nystatin
Integration into cell membrane disrupting membrane function.

Cell Wall

Mitochondrion

Plasma Membrane

(3) Azoles
Interruption of sterol biosynthesis (cell and mitochondrial membranes).

(4) Griseofulvin and
(5) 5-Fluorocytosine
Interruption of DNA and RNA synthesis.

Figure 11-2 Site of action of current antifungals.
1. Inhibition of cell wall synthesis → Echinocandins (capsofungin)
2. Membrane function → Amphotericin B and nystatin
3. Ergosterol synthesis → Azoles, allylamines
4. Nuclear division → Griseofulvin
5. Nucleic acid synthesis → Flucytosine

GENERAL CHARACTERISTICS OF IMIDAZOLES

Indications and Usage—Serious deep fungal infections and dermatological fungal infections caused by **Candida**, *Cryptococcus*, *Histoplasmosis*, *Blastomyces*, *Coccidioides*, and dermatophytes (*Epidermophyton*, *Microsporum*, and *Trichophyton*); *miconazole* and *clotrimazole* are commonly used for mucocutaneous (oropharyngeal, vaginal) candidiasis

Mechanism of Action—Binds **fungal cytochrome P450**, disrupting cell membrane function and increasing membrane permeability leading to cell lysis

Side Effects

- *Ketoconazole*: Hepatic toxicity, jaundice, **hemolytic anemia**
- *Itraconazole*: Idiosyncratic hepatitis
- *Fluconazole*: Rash, rarely Stevens-Johnson syndrome
- *Clotrimazole and miconazole*: Local irritation with erythema, burning, pruritus
- *Voriconazole*: Photophobia, altered color perception, increased liver enzymes, hallucinations

ANTIMYCOBACTERIALS

Rifampin, Isoniazid, Pyrazinamide, Ethambutol/Streptomycin—RIPE/S

Mycobacteria are rod-shaped, aerobic bacteria that are responsible for several serious diseases, including tuberculosis, leprosy, and a number of infections common in patients suffering from AIDS or other immunosuppressive disorders.

The most important disease caused by these bacteria (at least on your board exam) is tuberculosis. Recall that tuberculosis is a chronic disease that consists of multiple stages and is associated with weakness, fatigue, weight loss, and fever. Tuberculosis infections also involve the lungs and may give rise to chronic cough with hemoptysis. For the treatment of **active tuberculosis**, a four-drug regimen is recommended to prevent the emergence of drug resistance. This regimen consists of:

rifampin, isoniazid, pyrazinamide, ethambutol/streptomycin – **RIPE/S**

One of the most commonly tested (and clinically serious) side effects of these drugs is the occurrence of **hepatotoxicity** associated with *rifampin and isoniazid*.

HARDCORE

Fluconazole is the agent of choice for **Coccidioides meningitis**.

HARDCORE

Imidazoles also inhibit the human cytochrome P450 3A4 enzyme system. This can result in **increased** plasma concentrations of other drugs metabolized by this system, including *warfarin, benzodiazepines, HMG-CoA inhibitors*, and *digoxin*.

HARDCORE

Imidazoles are **fungicidal** and **broad-spectrum**.

HARDCORE

Ketoconazole causes testosterone levels to decrease by inhibiting adrenal steroid synthesis. This leads to **gynecomastia** in men and **menstrual irregularities** in women.

Drugs Used to Treat Tuberculosis

 Rifampin, isoniazid, pyrazinamide, ethambutol, streptomycin

RIFAMPIN

Indications and Usage

- Active and latent tuberculosis (TB) infections (*Mycobacterium* spp.)
- Prophylaxis against meningitis caused by *Neisseria* spp. and following exposure to *Haemophilus influenzae* type B
- Leprosy, in combination with *dapsone*

Mechanism of Action—***Inhibits bacterial RNA synthesis*** by binding to the β subunit of mycobacterial DNA-dependent RNA polymerase

Side Effects—***Hepatotoxicity***

ISONIAZID (INH)

Indications and Usage—Active and latent TB infections (*Mycobacterium* spp.). Also atypical infections caused by *Mycobacterium*, *M. bovis*, and *M. kansasii*

Mechanism of Action—***Inhibition of the synthesis of mycolic acid***, an important component of the mycobacterial cell wall

Side Effects—***Hepatotoxicity***, ***peripheral neuropathy***, agranulocytosis, aplastic anemia, and thrombocytopenia

- **INH**: Isoniazid causes Neuropathy and Hepatotoxicity

PYRAZINAMIDE

Indications and Usage—***Active tuberculosis*** infections only

Mechanism of Action—Unknown, but may involve inhibition of fatty acid synthetase I (FASI) of *M. tuberculosis*

Side Effects—Morbilliform rash, arthralgias, or myalgias. Inhibition of uric acid excretion can lead to hyperuricemia, but rarely leads to gout. Should not be used in women who are pregnant

ETHAMBUTOL

Indications and Usage—***Active TB infection only***. Also atypical *Mycobacterium*, *M. avium-intracellulare* complex, *M. bovis*, *M. kansasii*

Mechanism of Action—***Inhibition of mycobacterial arabinosyl transferases***, which are important in the synthesis of the essential cell wall component arabinoglycan

Side Effects—Retrobulbar neuritis, which leads to ***color blindness*** and optic neuritis

STREPTOMYCIN

An aminoglycoside antimicrobial.

Indications and Usage—Active and latent tuberculosis infections. Also, tularemia (caused by *Francisella tularensis*), plague (caused by *Yersinia pestis*), and in combination with tetracycline for brucellosis (caused by *Brucella abortus*); gram-negative bacteria

Mechanism of Action—Binds irreversibly to the ***30S subunit of the bacterial ribosome***, leading to inhibition of protein synthesis

Side Effects—Irreversible ***ototoxicity*** and reversible ***nephrotoxicity***

Drugs Used to Treat Leprosy

 Dapsone, clofazime

DAPSONE

Indications and Usage—Primarily used for ***leprosy*** (*Mycobacterium leprae*), usually in combination with *clofazimine* and *rifampin*

Mechanism of Action—***Inhibits bacterial folic acid synthesis***

Side Effects

- **Blood**: Hemolysis and ***methemoglobinemia***, dose-related and common
- **Skin:** Urticaria, erythema nodosum, erythema multiforme, Stevens-Johnson syndrome, and toxic epidermal necrolysis
- **GI:** Toxic hepatitis, leading to cholestatic jaundice

CLOFAZIMINE

Indications and Usage—Primarily for leprosy (*M. leprae*), usually in combination with *dapsone* and *rifampin*; atypical mycobacterial infections with *M. avium-intracellulare* complex, *M. bovis*, or *M. fortuitum*

Mechanism of Action

- **Antimicrobial action:** Unknown, but may involve inhibition of replication and growth of *Mycobacterium* spp. by **binding to mycobacterial DNA**
- **Anti-inflammatory action**: Enhancement of neutrophil and macrophage phagocytosis

Side Effects

- **GI:** GI distress, **bowel obstruction**
- **Skin**: Pink, red, brown, or black *skin discoloration*

 HARDCORE

Clofazimine may discolor bodily secretions, including tears, semen, urine, and sweat. Remember, *rifampin* and *pyrazinamide* also cause discoloration of bodily secretions.

ANTIVIRALS

 Drugs used to treat respiratory viral infections: *Amantadine, rimantadine, zanamivir, oseltamivir*

Drugs used to treat herpes infections: *Acyclovir, valacyclovir, penciclovir, famciclovir, valganciclovir, ganciclovir, cidofovir, foscarnet, idoxuridine, trifluridine*

Drugs used to treat hepatitis B and C infections: *Lamivudine, adefovir, ribavirin, interferon-α*

Drugs used to treat HIV infections: *Zidovudine (AZT), stavudine (d4T), didanosine (ddI), lamivudine (3TC), abacavir, zalcitabine (ddC), tenofovir, efavirenz, nevirapine, delavirdine, saquinavir, ritonavir, indinavir, nelfinavir, amprenavir, lopinavir, atazanavir, enfurvitide*

Viruses are the smallest infectious pathogen that afflicts humans. These tiny infectious units contain only one type of nucleic acid (RNA or DNA) and are enveloped with a protein coat that forms a capsid. While viruses are responsible for a vast number of different diseases, the pharmaceutical treatments available are relatively few. When tackling these drugs for the board exams, be sure to concentrate on both the different indications (type of tissue afflicted and viral type) and specific mechanism of action.

Drugs Used to Treat Respiratory Viral Infections

Amantadine, rimantadine, zanamivir, oseltamivir, ribavirin

Amantadine and Rimantadine

Indications and Usage—Prophylactic and symptomatic treatment of influenza A

Mechanism of Action—Unknown, but may involve **inhibition of viral uncoating**, a process necessary for infection after the influenza virus enters the host cell

Side Effects

- **Cardiovascular**: Heart failure, edema, orthostatic hypotension
- **CNS:** Nervousness, insomnia, dizziness, headache

HARDCORE

Also used for Parkinson's disease and drug-induced extra-pyramidal symptoms, because these agents increase the CNS release of dopamine.

Zanamivir and Oseltamivir

These drugs are neuraminidase inhibitors.

Indications and Usage—Prophylactic and symptomatic treatment of **influenza A and B**

Mechanism of Action—These agents **inhibit the active site of viral neuraminidase**, an enzyme responsible for **cleaving sialic acid residues** from carbohydrate moieties on the surfaces of both host cells and influenza virus envelopes. By inhibiting neuraminidase, viral aggregation occurs at the host cell surface (instead of within the host cell) and thereby reduces the amount of infectious virus released from the cell.

Side Effects—Nasal and throat discomfort, bronchospasm in patients with reactive airway disease

HARDCORE

Amantadine decreases the threshold for seizures.

HARDCORE

If neuraminidase inhibitors are started within 2 days after developing symptoms, these agents can reduce the duration of infection by decreasing viral shedding.

Drugs Used to Treat Herpes Infections

 Drugs used to treat herpes simplex virus (HSV) 1 and 2 and varicella-zoster virus (VZV) infections: *Acyclovir, valacyclovir, penciclovir, famciclovir*

Drugs used to treat cytomegalovirus (CMV) infections: *Ganciclovir, valganciclovir, foscarnet*

Ophthalmic antiherpetics: *Idoxuridine, trifluridine*

Drugs Used to Treat HSV/VZV Infections

Acyclovir, valacyclovir, penciclovir, famciclovir

Valacyclovir—**Prodrug of** *acyclovir*

Penciclovir—**Topical only**

Famciclovir—**Oral prodrug of** *penciclovir*

Acyclovir is the prototype drug in this class. It is an acyclic guanosine derivative prodrug that *requires intracellular conversion by viral and host enzymes to its active form*. The other drugs in this class have a similar mechanism of action but differ in their pharmacokinetic properties.

Indications and Usage

- Intravenous *acyclovir* is used in serious, disseminated HSV (type 1 or 2) or VZV infections.
- Oral *acyclovir* is used in mucosal and cutaneous HSV and VZV infections.
- *Valacyclovir* is used for prophylaxis against CMV in post-transplantation patients.

Mechanism of Action—**Thymidine kinase** is a viral enzyme that phosphorylates *acyclovir* monophosphate into *acyclovir* triphosphate. *Acyclovir* triphosphate acts as a **chain terminator** by incorporating into a growing viral DNA chain and ultimately results in the **inhibition of viral DNA polymerase**.

Side Effects—Usually well tolerated; rarely encephalopathy can occur

Drugs Used to Treat CMV Infections

Ganciclovir, valganciclovir, foscarnet

GANCICLOVIR AND VALGANCICLOVIR

Valganciclovir is a prodrug of *ganciclovir*.

Indications and Usage—CMV retinitis, colitis, or esophagitis. Also used prophylactically to **prevent CMV infection in transplant patients**

- **Gang** up on *CMV* with **Gan**ciclovir and Val**gan**ciclovir

Mechanism of Action—A chain terminator similar to *acyclovir*, except *ganciclovir* is more selective for the form of thymidine kinase encoded by CMV

Side Effects—Reversible bone marrow suppression, granulocytopenia, and thrombocytopenia

FOSCARNET

Indications and Usage—*Ganciclovir*-resistant CMV retinitis, *acyclovir*-resistant HSV infections, VZV infections

Mechanism of Action—An **inorganic pyrophosphate molecule** that inhibits viral DNA and RNA polymerase

Side Effects—Reversible renal dysfunction

Ophthalmic Antiherpetics

Idoxuridine, trifluridine

Indications and Usage—HSV keratitis

Mechanism of Action

- *Idoxuridine*: After being phosphorylated intracellularly to idoxuridine triphosphate, it is incorporated into the viral DNA, where it acts as a **chain terminator**, inhibiting DNA synthesis.
- *Trifluridine*: After being phosphorylated intracellularly to trifluridine triphosphate, it **inhibits viral thymidylate synthase**, blocking the conversion of dUMP to dTMP, and inhibiting viral DNA replication.

Side Effects—Ocular irritation

Drugs Used to Treat Hepatitis B and C

Drugs used to treat hepatitis B: *Lamivudine, adefovir, interferon-α*

Drugs used to treat hepatitis C: *Ribavirin, interferon-α*

Drugs Used to Treat Hepatitis B

Lamivudine, adefovir, interferon-α

LAMIVUDINE

This agent is an antiretroviral nucleoside analog.

HARDCORE

Foscarnet should not to be combined with other nephrotoxic drugs (e.g., *cyclosporine, amphotericin B, aminoglycosides*).

Indications and Usage—Retroviral infections, including HIV and hepatitis B virus (HBV)

Mechanism of Action—***Inhibits reverse transcriptase (RT)***, an enzyme necessary for conversion of viral RNA into DNA. Additionally, once inside the cell, it is converted to lamivudine triphosphate, which acts as a ***chain terminator*** by incorporating into a growing viral DNA strand.

Side Effects—Generally well tolerated. Pancreatitis can occur in children.

ADENFOVIR

Adenfovir is a reverse transcriptase inhibitor.

Indications and Usage—Infection with HBV

Mechanism of Action—Nucleotide reverse transcriptase inhibitor that interferes with viral RNA-dependent DNA polymerase, resulting in the inhibition of viral replication

Side Effects—Hematuria

Drugs Used to Treat Hepatitis C

 Ribavirin, interferon-α

RIBAVIRIN

This is a nucleoside analog.

Indications and Usage

- **RSV infections**: Inhaled *ribavirin* reduces morbidity in children with RSV bronchiolitis or pneumonia.
- **HCV infections**: Oral *ribavirin*, in combination with *interferon-α*, for the treatment of hepatitis C is more effective than interferon-α alone.
- Orthomyxoviridae, Paramyxoviridae, Arenaviridae

Mechanism of Action—*Ribavirin* is a ***nucleoside analog***, which inhibits the replication of RNA viruses through several mechanisms, including:

- Depletion of intracellular triphosphate pools secondary to inhibition of inosine monophosphate dehydrogenase
- Inhibition of the 5′-cap structure of viral mRNA
- Inhibition of virus-dependent RNA polymerases
- Alteration of the balance between proinflammatory and anti-inflammatory cytokines
- Induction of mutations in viral RNA

Side Effects—Oral *ribavirin* can produce hemolytic anemia, pruritus, and rash. Inhaled *ribavirin* can lead to dyspnea.

INTERFERON-α

Indications and Usage—Chronic hepatitis B infections, hepatitis D/hepatitis B coinfections, chronic hepatitis C infections

Mechanism of Action—***Interferon is a cytokine released by lymphocytes*** in response to viral infections and exerts its effect by:

1. Inhibiting viral replication
2. Increasing phagocytosis by immune cells
3. Increasing cytotoxicity of lymphocytes

Side Effects

- **General**: Flu-like syndrome with muscle aches, fatigue, fevers, and headaches
- **Hematologic**: Bone marrow suppression can lead to thrombocytopenia, neutropenia, and anemia.
- **Neurologic**: Depression, anxiety, emotional lability
- **Rheumatologic**: Autoimmune diseases may be induced or exacerbated

HARDCORE

Hepatitis D occurs only in patients infected with hepatitis B virus.

HARDCORE

Interferon alpha is used in combination with *ribavirin* for the treatment of hepatitis C.

Drugs Used to Treat HIV Infections

 Nucleoside reverse transcriptase inhibitors (NRTIs): *AZT, stavudine, didanosine, lamivudine, abacavir, zalcitabine*

Nucleotide reverse transcriptase inhibitors (NtRTIs): *Tenofovir*

Non-nucleoside reverse transcriptase inhibitors (NNRTIs): *Efavirenz, nevirapine, delavirdine*

Protease inhibitors (PIs): *Saquinavir, ritonavir, indinavir, nelfinavir, amprenavir, lopinavir, atazanavir*

Viral entry inhibitors: *Enfurvitide*

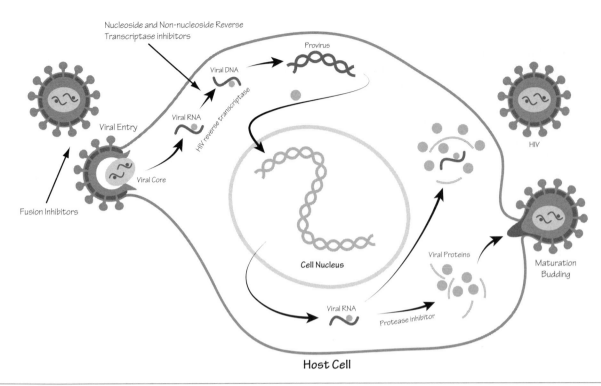

Figure 11-3 Sites of action of antiretroviral therapy. Fusion inhibitors block the entry of the virus into cells. Reverse transcriptase inhibitors (NRTIs and NNRTIs) prevent the conversion of HIV viral RNA strand into the DNA strand necessary for the ability of the virus to infect the cell. Protease inhibitors block the viral protease that cleaves viral polypeptide protein into functional protein, which is required for production of viable HIV particles.

HIV is a retrovirus that attacks lymphocytes and other cells expressing the CD4 surface protein. HIV gradually depletes the body of CD4+ lymphocytes, creating an ideal environment for opportunistic pathogens. As the disease progresses and the CD4 count drops, the infected individual may eventually succumb to any number of infectious organisms. Drugs currently used in the treatment of HIV have three targets: HIV entry (fusion inhibitors), HIV reverse transcriptase, and HIV protease. The enzyme reverse transcriptase enables HIV to convert its own RNA into DNA for subsequent incorporation into the host cell genome, allowing for massive replication of the virus. The viral protease enzyme is essential for cleaving polyproteins and generating specific proteins necessary to form mature and functional viruses, the final step of viral proliferation.

Basic Principles of HIV Therapy

Remember, *there is no cure for HIV*.

1. Recommendations for initiating therapy:
   - Symptomatic HIV (e.g., opportunistic infections)
   - Asymptomatic HIV with < 200 CD4 cells/μL
   - Asymptomatic HIV with > 200 CD4 cells/μL. Recommendations are based on CD4 count and rate of decline and HIV RNA level in the plasma.
2. Therapy should consist of at least a ***three-drug regimen***.
3. Classes of anti-HIV drugs include:
   - NRTIs, NtRTIs, and NNRTIs, the inhibitors of the viral enzyme ***reverse transcriptase***
   - Inhibitors of the viral ***protease enzyme*** (PIs)
   - Inhibitors of ***viral entry*** into CD4 cells

NUCLEOSIDE REVERSE TRANSCRIPTASE INHIBITORS (NRTIS)

 Zidovudine (AZT)**, stavudine **(d4T)**, didanosine **(ddI)**, lamivudine **(3TC)**, abacavir, zalcitabine **(ddC)

Mechanism of Action—***Inhibit reverse transcriptase***, the enzyme responsible for the conversion of viral RNA into DNA. Additionally, once inside the cell NRTIs are phosphorylated and incorporated into the growing HIV DNA strand, and causing chain termination.

Side Effects

- *Zidovudine*: Anemia, neutropenia, hepatitis
- *Stavudine, didanosine, lamivudine, zalcitabine*: Dose-related peripheral sensory neuropathy, pancreatitis
- *Abacavir*: Severe hypersensitivity reaction in 5% of patients

Nucleotide Reverse Transcriptase Inhibitors (NtRTIs)

 Tenofovir

Mechanism of Action—Nucleotides are phosphorylated nucleosides, which inhibit reverse transcriptase and cause chain termination in a similar fashion to the NRTIs

Side Effects—Muscular weakness

Non-Nucleoside Reverse Transcriptase Inhibitors (NNRTIs)

 Efavirenz, nevirapine, delavirdine

The "**-vir**" drugs.

Mechanism of Action—NNRTIs are similar to NRTIs because they **inhibit HIV reverse transcriptase**. However, the mechanisms of reverse transcriptase inhibition differ—NNRTIs bind to a non-enzymatic portion of reverse transcriptase, leading to a **conformational change in the enzyme** and rendering it inactive.

Side Effects

- *Efavirenz*: CNS disturbances (insomnia, nightmares, hallucinations)
- *Nevirapine*: Hepatotoxicity, possibly leading to hepatic failure and death

HARDCORE

NNRTI inhibition of reverse transcriptase is an example of *allosteric* inhibition.

Protease Inhibitors (PIs)

 Saquinavir, ritonavir, indinavir, nelfinavir, amprenavir, lopinavir, atazanavir

The "-navir" drugs.

Mechanism of Action—PIs **inhibit the enzyme HIV protease**. HIV protease normally cleaves precursor proteins into the individual components necessary for HIV maturation, infectivity, and replication.

Side Effects

- When thinking of side effects for PIs, associate them with the **diet of the typical American patient**: Hyperglycemia secondary to insulin resistance and hyperlipidemia
- **Cushingoid-like appearance**: Associated with fat redistribution and accumulation around the stomach, upper back, and face with fat wasting on the upper and lower extremities
- Kidney stones, primarily with *indinavir*
- All are associated with hepatotoxicity, primarily *ritonavir*

HARDCORE

The most common side effects of the PIs are gastrointestinal disturbances, including *diarrhea, nausea, and vomiting*.

Viral Entry Inhibitors (Fusion Inhibitors)

 Enfurvitide

Mechanism of Action—*Enfurvitide inhibits the fusion of the HIV-1 virus with CD4 cells* by blocking the conformational change of the viral envelope glycoprotein gp41 subunits, which are required for membrane fusion and entry into CD4 cells.

Side Effects—Insomnia; local injection site irritation is also common

ANTIPARASITICS

 Antimalarials: *Primaquine, chloroquine, quinine, quinidine, mefloquine, proguanil, pyrimethamine*
Anticestodes: *Niclosamide*
Antiflagellates: *Metronidazole, nifurtimox, suramin, pentavalent antimony*
Antinematodes: *Ivermectin, mebendazole, pyrantel pamoate, thiabendazole*
Antitrematodes: *Praziquantel*

Parasitology encompasses a wide variety of infectious diseases and organisms, most of which are fairly uncommon in the United States. This is probably the reason that the board exam tends to not include a large number of questions on these drugs.

Antimalarials

 Primaquine, chloroquine, quinine, mefloquine, proguanil, pyrimethamine

Malaria is a disease caused by the parasite genus *Plasmodium*, and is transmitted to humans through the bite of the female *Anopheles* mosquito. Infections by *Plasmodium* can vary in severity depending on the species of the parasite, but generally include fever, hypotension, erythrocytosis, and possibly death. Antimalarial agents target stages in the life cycle of the malarial parasite (Figure 11-4).

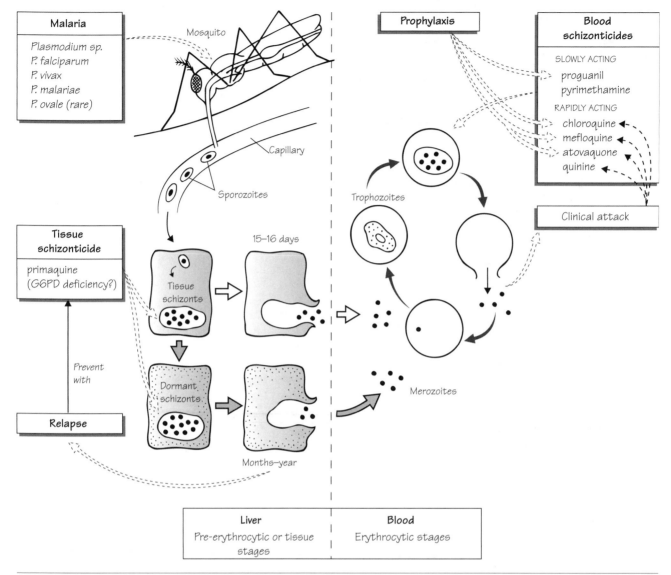

Figure 11-4 Antimalarials. Malaria is caused by four species of protozoa that have part of their life cycle in the female *Anopheles* mosquito. These protozoa enter human circulation via a mosquito bite and are carried to the liver, where they multiply and form tissue schizonts. After 5 to 16 d, the schizonts rupture and release thousands of merozoites that infect red blood cells, initiating the malarial erythrocytic stage. Most antimalarials are **blood schizonticides** and are toxic to the erythrocytic schizonts. *Primaquine* is a **tissue schizonticide** and is effective at eliminating schizonts within the liver. (Reprinted with permission from Neal MJ. Medical Pharmacology at a Glance. 4th ed. Oxford: Blackwell Publishing, 2002:90.)

HARDCORE

Primaquine should not be given to patients with glucose-6-phosphate dehydrogenase deficiency due to a risk of **drug-induced hemolytic anemia.**

HARDCORE

Resistance to *chloroquine* is becoming increasingly common and has caused its use to be limited in certain geographical locations, especially Asia and some areas of Central and South America.

HARDCORE

Chloroquine is also occasionally used in rheumatoid arthritis and discoid lupus erythematosus due to its anti-inflammatory actions.

PRIMAQUINE
A tissue schizonticide.

Indications and Usage—Infections due to primary and secondary forms of *Plasmodium*, but **not** erythrocytic schizonts

Mechanism of Action—Intermediates from these drugs oxidize reduced glutathione, **depleting antioxidant molecules and allowing toxic free radicals to accumulate.**

Side Effects—Granulocytopenia

CHLOROQUINE
A blood schizonticide.

Indications and Usage—Erythrocytic malaria

Mechanism of Action—Chloroquine **enters RBCs and inhibits proteinases** in food vacuoles, allowing soluble heme in the cell to accumulate, which is toxic to the parasite. Additionally, chloroquine **decreases parasitic DNA synthesis** by disrupting the tertiary structure of nucleic acids.

Side Effects—Rash, nightmares, visual disturbances, chronic nail bed discoloration

QUININE AND MEFLOQUINE
A blood schizonticide.

Indications and Usage—Malarial strains resistant to other drugs

Mechanism of Action—Depresses parasite oxygen uptake and carbohydrate metabolism, and intercalates into DNA, disrupting parasite replication and transcription

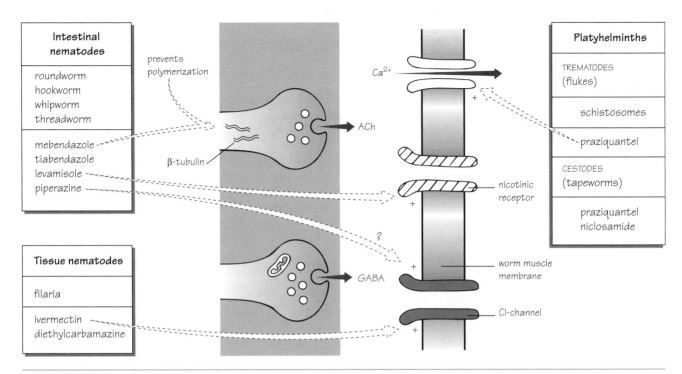

Figure 11-5 Drugs acting on parasites. Helminths are worms that are either round (nematodes) or flat (platyhelminths). The nervous systems of these organisms differ from those in vertebrates, providing the point of attack for most antiparasitic medications. (Reprinted with permission from Neal MJ. Medical Pharmacology at a Glance. 4th ed. Oxford: Blackwell Publishing, 2002:88.)

Side Effects—***Cinchonism***: nausea, vomiting, tinnitus, vertigo; possible cardiac arrest and ECG abnormalities

PROGUANIL AND PYRIMETHAMINE
Blood schizonticides.

Indications and Usage—Prophylaxis for malaria

Mechanism of Action—Act as ***folate antagonists*** that inhibit dihydrofolate reductase, resulting in the inhibiting of DNA synthesis and cell division

Side Effects—Rash, GI distress, pruritus

Anticestodes

 Niclosamide

Indications and Usage—Tapeworm infections (*Diphyllobothrium latum* and *Taenia* spp.)

Mechanism of Action—Inhibits parasite anaerobic phosphorylation of ADP in mitochondria

Side Effects—Nausea and abdominal pain

Antiflagellates

 Metronidazole, nifurtimox, suramin

METRONIDAZOLE

Indications and Usage—*Giardia*, *Entamoeba histolytica* (amebic dysentery), bacteria vaginitis (*Gardnerella vaginalis*), *Trichomonas*, *Clostridium difficile* (pseudomembranous colitis)

Mechanism of Action—Forms reduced ***cytotoxic compounds that bind parasitic proteins and DNA***, resulting in death of the parasite

Side Effects—GI distress, ***disulfiram reaction with alcohol***

NIFURTIMOX

Indications and Usage—*Trypanosoma cruzi* (**Chagas' disease**)

Mechanism of Action—***Generates intracellular oxygen radicals*** that are toxic to the parasite

Side Effects—Anaphylaxis, peripheral neuropathy, immunosuppression

SURAMIN

Indications and Usage—African trypanosomiasis (sleeping sickness)

Mechanism of Action—Inhibits enzymes involved in parasitic energy metabolism

Side Effects—Primarily renal, including albuminuria, hematuria, and casts

HARDCORE

Proguanil and *pyrimethamine* are used to prevent malarial infection because they have 1000 times the affinity for the plasmodial enzyme than for the human enzyme.

HARDCORE

Niclosamide is lethal for the cestode scolex and segments, but not for ova.

Antinematodes

 Ivermectin, mebendazole

IVERMECTIN

Indications and Usage—*Onchocera volvulus* (river blindness)

Mechanism of Action—*Ivermectin* enhances chloride efflux by increasing **parasite GABA receptor activation**, resulting in paralysis of the worm.

Side Effects—Hypotension, dizziness

MEBENDAZOLE

Indications and Usage—Whipworm, hookworm, pinworm, and roundworm infections

Mechanism of Action—**Interferes with parasite synthesis of microtubules**

Side Effects—Not absorbed with oral ingestion resulting in limited side effects

Antitrematodes

 Praziquantel

Indications and Usage—Trematode infections

Mechanism of Action—Increases permeability of the parasitic cell membrane to calcium, causing paralysis of the parasite

Side Effects—GI distress, drug interactions

HARDCORE

Praziquantel is contraindicated in the treatment of ocular cysticercosis because destruction of the worm in the eye may damage ocular function.

HARDCORE REVIEW – ANTIFUNGAL, ANTIMYCOBACTERIAL, ANTIVIRAL, AND ANTIPARASITIC PHARMACOLOGY

TABLE 11-1 Antifungals

DRUG CLASS	DRUGS	HARDCORE BUG TARGETS	MECHANISM OF ACTION	MAJOR SIDE EFFECTS
Subcutaneous and systemic antifungals	Amphotericin B	• Candida • Cryptococcus • Histoplasmosis • Blastomyces • Coccidioides • Aspergillus	Binds fungal cell ergosterol forming membrane pores. *Fungicidal*	Nephrotoxicity, hypotension, anemia, thrombophlebitis
	Caspofungin	• Aspergillus • Candida	Inhibition of β-1,3 glucan synthase	Pruritus bronchospasm
	Flucytosine	• Chromomycoses • Candida • Cryptococcus • Aspergillus	Pyrimidine antimetabolite, converted to 5-FdUMP that inhibits thymidylate synthase and the production of DNA. *Fungicidal*	Neutropenia, thrombocytopenia due to *bone marrow suppression*
	Terbinafine	• Onychomycoses • Dermatophytes	Blocks ergosterol synthesis by inhibiting squalene epoxidase *Fungicidal*	Loss of taste
Superficial antifungals	Nystatin	• Candidiasis	Binds to ergosterol, disrupts fungal membranes altering permeability and leading to cell lysis	Rare topically
	Griseofulvin	• Dermatophyte infections • Tinea capitis	Inhibits fungal microtubule function	Pancytopenia
	Naftifine	• Dermatophyte onychomycoses	Inhibits squalene epoxidase/fungal sterol biosynthesis	Neutropenia, lymphopenia
Imidazoles – General and topical	Clotrimazole, miconazole, ketoconazole	• Candida • Cryptococcus • Histoplasmosis • Blastomyces • Coccidioides • Dermatophytes	Inhibits fungal cytochrome P450 *Fungicidal*	Local irritation
Systemic imidazoles	Fluconazole	• Coccidiodes	Inhibits fungal cytochrome P450 *Fungicidal*	Stevens-Johnson syndrome
	Itraconazole	• Aspergillus		Idiosyncratic hepatitis
	Ketoconazole	• Candida		*Gynecomastia*, hepatic toxicity
	Voriconazole	• Aspergillus		Blurred vision, photophobia, altered color perception

TABLE 11-2 Antimycobacterium

Drug Class	Drugs	Hardcore Bug Targets	Mechanism of Action	Major Side Effects
Anti-tuberculosis	Rifampin	• *M. tuberculosis* • *M. leprae* • *Neisseria* • *H. influenzae* type B	*Inhibits bacterial RNA by binding mycobaterial DNA-dependent RNA polymerase; Bactericidal*	Hepatotoxicity, body secretion discoloration
	Isoniazid	• *M. tuberculosis* • *M. bovis* • *M. kansasii*	Inhibits the synthesis of mycolic acid; *bactericidal*	Hepatotoxicity and peripheral neuropathy
	Pyrazinamide	• *M. tuberculosis*	Inhibits fatty acid synthetase I (FASI) of *M. tuberculosis*; *bactericidal*	Hyperuricemia, body secretion discoloration
	Ethambutol	• *M. tuberculosis* • *M. avium-intracellulare* • *M. bovis* • *M. kansasii*	Inhibits cell wall *arabinogalactan*; *bacteriostatic*	Color blindness
	Streptomycin	• *M. tuberculosis* • Gram (-) enterics • *Pseudomonas* • *Francisella tularensis* • *Yersinia pestis* • *Brucella abortus*	Binds the 30S subunit of the bacterial ribosome	Ototoxicity, nephrotoxicity
Anti-leprosy	Dapsone	• *M. leprae*	Inhibits bacterial folic acid synthesis	Methemoglobinemia, erythema multiforme
	Clofazimine	• *M. leprae* • *M. avium-complex* • *M. bovis* • *M fortuitum*	Binds and inhibits mycobacterial DNA replication, enhances immuno-phagocytosis	Bowel obstruction, skin discoloration

TABLE 11-3 Antivirals: Respiratory, Anti-HSV/VZV, Anti-CMV, Ophthalmic Antiherpetics, Anti-Hepatitis

Drug Class	Drugs	Hardcore Bug Targets	Mechanism of Action	Major Side Effects
Respiratory antivirals	Amantadine, rimantadine	• **Influenza A**	Inhibits viral uncoating	Seizures, heart failure, orthostatic hypotension
	Zanamivir, oseltamivir	• Influenza A and B	Inhibits neuraminidase	Bronchospasm in asthmatics
	Ribavirin	• Respiratory syncytial virus (RSV) • HCV • Orthomyxoviridae • Paramyxoviridae • Arenaviridae	A nucleoside analog that inhibits the replication of RNA viruses	Hemolytic anemia, dyspnea
• Anti-herpes simplex virus (HSV) 1 and 2 • Anti-varicella-zoster virus (VZV)	Acyclovir, valacyclovir, penciclovir, famciclovir	• HSV • VZV • CMV prophylaxis for post-transplant patients with valacyclovir	Activated by thymidine kinase, ultimately inhibits viral DNA polymerase	Rarely encephalopathy with seizures
Anti-cytomegalovirus (CMV)	Ganciclovir, valganciclovir	• CMV	Specific to thymidine kinase encoded by CMV, inhibits viral DNA polymerase	Bone marrow suppression, granulocytopenia, thrombocytopenia
	Foscarnet	• CMV • HSV • VZV	Acts as an inorganic pyrophosphate molecule inhibiting viral DNA and RNA polymerase	Nephrotoxicity
	Cidofovir	• CMV	Acts as a cytosine nucleotide analog, leading to viral DNA chain termination	Nephrotoxicity
Ophthalmic antiherpetics	Idoxuridine	• HSV	Incorporated into viral DNA, leading to chain termination	Eye irritation
	Trifluridine	• HSV	Inhibits viral thymidylate synthase conversion of dUMP to dTMP, inhibiting viral DNA replication	Eye irritation
Anti-hepatitis	Lamivudine	• HIV • HBV	Inhibits RT, causes chain termination by incorporating into the growing viral DNA	Rarely pancreatitis in children
	Adefovir	• HBV	Reverse transcriptase inhibitor, interferes with HBV viral RNA dependent DNA polymerase	Hematuria
	Interferon-α	• HBV • HCV • HDV	Inhibits viral replication, increases immunophagocytosis, increases cytotoxicity of lymphocytes	Flu-like symptoms, depression, bone marrow suppression

TABLE 11-4 Antivirals: HIV

Drug Class	Drugs	Hardcore Bug Targets	Mechanism of Action	Major Side Effects
Nucleoside reverse transcriptase inhibitors (NRTIs) the "-vudine" drugs	Zidovudine (AZT), stavudine, didanosine, lamivudine, abacavir, zalcitabine	HIV	Inhibits RT, incorporated into growing the HIV DNA leading to chain termination	Lactic acidosis **Zidovudine:** Anemia, neutropenia, hepatitis **Zalcitabine:** Peripheral neuropathy, pancreatitis **Abacavir:** Hypersensitivity reaction
Nucleotide reverse transcriptase inhibitors (NtRTIs)	Tenofovir	HIV	Inhibits HIV reverse transcriptase	Muscular weakness
Non-nucleoside reverse transcriptase inhibitors (NNRTIs) the "-vir-" drugs	Efavirenz, nevirapine, delavirdine	HIV	Inhibits HIV RT by conformational change	Insomnia, hepatotoxicity
Protease inhibitors the "-navir" drugs	Saquinavir, ritonavir, indinavir, nelfinavir, amprenavir, lopinavir, atazanavir	HIV	Inhibits HIV protease	Cushingoid-like appearance, hepatotoxicity, kidney stones
Viral entry inhibitors	Enfurvitide	HIV	Inhibits fusion of HIV-1 with CD4 cells	Insomnia

TABLE 11-5 Antiparasitics

Drug Class	Drugs	Hardcore Bug Targets	Mechanism of Action	Major Side Effects
Antimalarials	Primaquine	• Plasmodium tissue schizonticide	Oxidizes reduced glutathione	Granulocytopenia
	Chloroquine	• Plasmodium blood schizonticide (erythrocytic malaria)	**Inhibits RBCs, allowing the accumulation of soluble heme; decreases parasitic DNA synthesis**	Nightmares, nail bed discoloration
	Quinine, mefloquine	• Plasmodium blood schizonticide	Depresses parasitic oxygen/carbohydrate uptake and metabolism; disrupts parasitic replication and transcription	Cinchonism
	Proguanil, primethamine	• Plasmodium blood schizonticide	**Folate antagonists** that inhibit dihydrofolate reductase	Rash, GI distress, pruritus
Anticestodes	Niclosamide	Tapeworm infections • D. latum • Taenia species	Inhibits parasitic anaerobic phosphorylation of ADP in mitochondria	
Antiflagellates	Metronidazole	• Giardia • Amebic dysentery • G. vaginalis • Trichomonas • Clostridium difficile	Forms reduced cytotoxic compounds that bind and are toxic to parasitic proteins and DNA	Disulfiram reaction with alcohol
	Nifurtimox	• T. cruzi	Generates intracellular oxygen radicals	Anaphylaxis, neuropathy
	Suramin	• African trypanosomiasis (sleeping sickness)	Inhibits enzymes involved in parasitic energy metabolism	Renal toxicity
Antinematodes	Ivermectin	• O. volvulus (river blindness)	Increasing parasitic GABA receptor activation	Hypotension, dizziness
	Mebendazole	• Whipworm • Hookworm • Pinworm • Roundworm	Interferes with parasite synthesis of microtubules	Rare
	Pyrantel pamoate	• Roundworms • Pinworms • Hookworms	Depolarizes parasite neuromuscular nicotinic receptors	GI distress
	Thiabendazole	• Trichinella • S. stercoralis (threadworm)	Interferes with parasitic microtubular aggregation	Erythema multiforme, Stevens-Johnson syndrome
Antitrematodes	Praziquantel	• Trematodes	Increases permeability of the parasitic cell membrane to calcium, causing paralysis	GI distress

CHAPTER 12

Toxicology

Toxicology is the study of the effects and treatment of poisonous substances in biological systems. The following definitions are commonly used in the field of toxicology:

- **Poisons**: Any agent capable of producing a deleterious or deadly effect on a biological system. This definition, interpreted broadly, encompasses every known chemical. Every chemical is toxic given the right amount.
  - ○ Remember, **the dose** determines whether or not a chemical will cause a toxic response.
- **Toxins**: Toxic substances produced by biological systems
- **Toxicants**: Toxic substances produced as a result of human activities

The board exam will expect you to be familiar with the toxic compounds outlined in this chapter, and the treatment, or antidote, for each.

- Common drugs: *Acetaminophen, ethanol (alcohol), ethyl glycol, methanol, aspirin, atropine, barbiturates, benzodiazepines, digitalis, fibrinolytic drugs, heparin, opiates*
- Heavy metals: *Arsenic, iron, lead, mercury*
- Insecticides: *Organophosphorus compounds, carbamates, chlorinated hydrocarbons, botanical insecticides*
- Herbicides: *Bipyridyl herbicides (paraquat)*
- Rodenticides: *Sodium fluoroacetate, strychnine, warfarin*
- Air pollutants: *Carbon monoxide (CO), sulfur oxides, nitrogen oxides*

TOXIC SIDE EFFECTS OF COMMONLY USED DRUGS

Any pharmacological agent used in excess can become a poison. The following are commonly used therapeutic agents that have known toxic side effects:

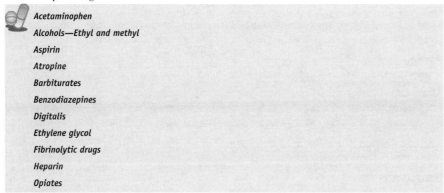

Acetaminophen
Alcohols—Ethyl and methyl
Aspirin
Atropine
Barbiturates
Benzodiazepines
Digitalis
Ethylene glycol
Fibrinolytic drugs
Heparin
Opiates

Acetaminophen

Mechanism of Toxicity—*Acetaminophen* is normally broken down in the liver to the **toxic intermediate N-acetyl-benzoquinoneimine (NAPQI)**. With normal doses, NAPQI reacts with the antioxidant **glutathione** to form a nontoxic metabolite that is subsequently excreted. However, in the presence of excessive *acetaminophen* levels, available hepatic glutathione stores are depleted, thereby allowing excess NAPQI to react with hepatic proteins and lipids, ultimately resulting in **centrilobular necrosis**.

Toxic Effects—Hepatic and renal tubular necrosis

Treatment—Restoration of glutathione stores with **N-acetylcysteine (NAC)**. NAC is a thiol antioxidant capable of both reducing oxidized glutathione and directly binding toxic free radicals.

Ethanol ("Booze" or Ethyl Alcohol)

Mechanism of Toxicity—Ethanol is converted to *acetaldehyde* by alcohol dehydrogenase and cytochrome P450 in the liver that is capable of covalently binding proteins and other macromolecules.

Toxic Effects—Nausea, vomiting, headache, hypotension, CNS depression

Treatment—Fluids, symptomatic treatment, and withdrawal prophylaxis (*benzodiazepines*); dialysis if necessary

Methanol (Methyl Alcohol, Varnish)

Mechanism of Toxicity—*Methanol* is metabolized in the liver by alcohol dehydrogenase (ADH) to *formaldehyde*, which is subsequently converted to *formic acid*. Formic acid, which is normally broken down to carbon dioxide, is directly toxic in excessive amounts.

Toxic Effects—*Retinal damage*, metabolic acidosis

Treatment—Administration of *ethanol or 4-methylpyrazole* (an ADH inhibitor), which compete with methanol for ADH binding sites, and thereby decrease the formation of formic acid. Also, sodium bicarbonate to correct metabolic acidosis

Aspirin (Salicylates)

Mechanism of Toxicity—Salicylates uncouple cellular oxidative phosphorylation and, with elevated levels, may result in respiratory depression following a period of respiratory stimulation. This eventually leads to a combination of *uncompensated respiratory and metabolic acidosis*.

Toxic Effects—Uncompensated respiratory and metabolic acidosis, hyperthermia

Treatment—Salicylates are organic acids, so alkalizing the urine keeps the salicylate molecules in a charged state and concentrates them in the urine for excretion. Dialysis can be used as a last resort.

Atropine

Mechanism of Toxicity—Nonselective blockade of muscarinic acetylcholine receptors

Toxic Effects—Remember this mnemonic, which describes the symptoms of muscarinic receptor blockage:

- **Blind as a bat**—Blocks the ability of the pupil to constrict, resulting in mydriasis and the inability to focus for near vision (cycloplegia)
- **Mad as a hatter**—Acts in the CNS causing restlessness, confusion, and delirium
- **Dry as a bone**—Blocks salivary, lacrimal, and sweat gland secretions
- **Hot as hell**—Elevates body temperature
- **Red as a beet**—Causes dilation of the cutaneous vasculature, likely due to the elevation in body temperature

Treatment—Since atropine competitively blocks muscarinic receptors, its effect can be overcome by increasing the amount of acetylcholine present. For this reason, administration of the acetylcholinesterase inhibitor, *physostigmine*, is used to treat atropine poisoning.

Barbiturates

 Phenobarbital, pentobarbital, thiopental

Mechanism of Toxicity—Excessive GABA-mediated CNS depression

Toxic Effects—Severe respiratory and cardiovascular depression

Treatment—*No specific antidote*; mechanical ventilation along with gastric lavage and alkalinization of the urine for enhanced excretion

Benzodiazepines

 Diazepam, lorazepam, midazolam, chlordiazepoxide, triazolam, oxazepam

Mechanism of Toxicity—Excessive GABA-mediated CNS depression

Toxic Effects—Respiratory depression

Treatment—Administration of *flumazenil*, a competitive antagonist at GABA receptors, can reverse the effects of a benzodiazepine overdose.

Digitalis

Mechanism of Toxicity—Digitalis acts by inhibiting the membrane-bound Na^+/K^+-ATPase enzyme that normally pumps sodium out of, and potassium into, myocardial cells. Inhibition of this transporter results in a *decreased intracellular potassium level and an increased intracellular sodium level*. Also, *an increase in intracellular calcium level* occurs due to the decreased activity of the Na^+-Ca^{2+} exchanger in the presence of high levels of intracellular Na^+.

Toxic Effects—Arrhythmias, nausea, vomiting, diarrhea, abdominal pain, dizziness, confusion, delirium, electrolyte abnormalities (these effects can be even more profound in the presence of serum hypokalemia)

Treatment—Administration of *digoxin-immune Fab*, an antibody that binds *digoxin*, which then is excreted in the urine. Potassium normalization; arrhythmia treatment with *lidocaine*

Ethylene Glycol (Antifreeze)

Mechanism of Toxicity—Ethylene glycol is ultimately converted to glyoxylic acid by a series of reactions. Glyoxylic acid may then be metabolized to either *oxalic acid or formic acid*, both of which are directly toxic.

Toxic Effects—An asymptomatic period following ingestion gives way to period of inebriation, metabolic acidosis (due to an accumulation of oxalic acid), tachycardia, and tachypnea that occurs approximately 24 hours after ingestion and can progress to cardiac failure and pulmonary edema. Renal toxicity occurs 1 to 3 days after ingestion.

Treatment—Administration of *ethanol or 4-methylpyrazole* (an ADH inhibitor) to minimize the number of ADH binding sites available for the conversion of ethylene glycol to its toxic metabolites; sodium bicarbonate administration to treat the metabolic acidosis

Fibrinolytic Drugs

Alteplase (tPA), streptokinase, urokinase

Mechanism of Toxicity—These fibrinolytic agents convert plasminogen bound to fibrin, within a clot, to plasmin. Plasmin then cleaves fibrin, resulting in lysis of the thrombus.

Toxic Effects—*Excessive bleeding* from an increased rate of fibrinolysis

Treatment—*Aminocaproic acid*, which blocks the binding of plasminogen and plasmin to fibrin

Heparin

Mechanism of Toxicity—*Binds antithrombin III*, which acts to prevent thrombin from converting fibrinogen to fibrin. Also binds and *inhibits coagulation factor Xa*

Toxic Effects—Excessive bleeding due to anticoagulant effect of heparin

Treatment—Administration of *protamine sulfate*

Opiates

Mechanism of Toxicity—Opioid receptor-mediated CNS depression

Toxic Effects—CNS and respiratory depression

Treatment—The opiate antagonists *naloxone* or *naltrexone*. These agents act as pure opioid antagonists that compete and displace opiates at opioid receptor sites.

HEAVY METALS

Heavy metals are common in the environment; however, excessive exposure may lead to serious toxic effects. Typically, heavy metal toxicity is treated with a chelating medication that binds the metal and enables the complex to be excreted. The following are some important toxic heavy metals:

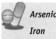
Arsenic
Iron
Lead
Mercury

ARSENIC

Mechanism of Toxicity—Binds sulfhydryl groups on proteins and interferes with numerous enzyme systems, including those involved in cellular respiration, gluconeogenesis, glucose uptake, and glutathione metabolism

Toxic Effects—Acute and chronic exposure to arsenic may cause:

- **Gastrointestinal**: *Nausea*, vomiting, diarrhea
- **Cardiovascular/pulmonary**: Hypotension, metabolic acidosis, *pulmonary edema, arrhythmias*, peripheral vascular disease chronically
- **Neurologic**: Delirium, coma, *ascending sensorimotor peripheral neuropathy*
- **Hematologic**: Massive intravascular *hemolysis*, jaundice

HARDCORE

Some patients suffering from digitalis toxicity present complaining of disturbed color perception and report seeing everything in shades of blue and green. This is called the *"digitalis aura."*

HARDCORE

Chelation of calcium by oxalic acid results in the formation of *calcium oxalate crystals*. Precipitation of these crystals in the renal tubules is involved in the nephrotoxicity associated with ethylene glycol.

- **Dermatologic**: Hyperpigmentation of skin, hyperkeratoses on the palms and soles, *Mees lines* (horizontal white bands on finger nails)
- **Genitourinary**: Hemoglobinuria, increased incidence of bladder cancer and renal failure

Treatment—Chelation therapy using *dimercaprol (BAL) or succimer*

IRON

Mechanism of Toxicity—Progressive iron accumulation in hepatic, pancreatic, cardiac, and skin tissues results in cellular dysfunction

Toxic Effects—Liver dysfunction, heart failure, skin pigmentation, and diabetes mellitus

Treatment—Chelation therapy using *deferoxamine*

LEAD

Mechanism of Toxicity—Inhibits various enzymes and alters the structure of cell membranes; interferes with the action of cations such as calcium, iron, and zinc

Toxic Effects

- **Acute toxic effects** include thirst and a metallic taste in the mouth, as well as abdominal pain and milky vomit; shock can occur following ingestion of large amounts of lead due to osmotic movement of large amounts of water into the gut; muscle weakness; nephrotoxicity
  - If the patient survives acute intoxication, chronic toxic effects may become apparent.
- **Chronic toxic effects** are more common in children than adults, and include
  - **Neurologic**: Neurocognitive impairment in children such as fatigue, *sleep disturbance, slowed reaction time*; adults are less sensitive, but may still display neurocognitive effects especially *peripheral neuropathy and memory loss*; acute exposure to organolead compounds, such as those found in leaded gasoline, can result in severe CNS effects, including hallucinations, delirium, and convulsions
  - **Hematologic**: *Anemia* due to inhibition of heme synthesis and decreased red cell survival time
  - **Renal/CV**: Chronic exposure can result in *nephrosclerosis*; *hypertension* can occur due to changes in vascular smooth muscle tone
  - **Dental**: *Lead lines* on gingivae
  - **Skeletal**: Lead lines on epiphyses of long bones

Treatment—Remove the patient from the source of exposure; chelation therapy with *dimercaprol* or *calcium disodium EDTA* (CaNa$_2$ EDTA); supportive care

MERCURY

Mechanism of Toxicity—Inhibition of enzymatic activity and alteration of membrane function due to interaction with sulfhydryl groups

Toxic Effects

- **Inhaled vapor**: Acute inhalation exposure results in *gingivostomatitis*, pneumonitis, and pulmonary edema; chronic exposure results in tremor (also choreiform movements), *neuropsychiatric disturbances* (memory loss, insomnia, mood changes), and gingivostomatitis.
- **Oral ingestion**: Hemorrhagic gastroenteritis and renal failure

Treatment—Chelation therapy using *dimercaprol (BAL)* or *succimer*

INSECTICIDES

There are several types of insecticides that may appear on Step 1. These include:

Organophosphorus compounds
Carbamates
Organochlorine compounds
Botanical insecticides

Organophosphorus Compounds

Diisopropylflurophosphate (DFP), nerve gases, malathion

Mechanism of Toxicity—Covalent inhibition of the enzyme acetylcholinesterase

Toxic Effects—Excessive cholinergic stimulation at nicotinic and muscarinic receptors. These effects include **SLUDE** *(Salivation, Lacrimation, Urination, Defecation, and Emesis)* **syndrome**, bronchoconstriction and increased bronchosecretions, muscular fasciculations, and, in severe cases, *paralysis and death due to respiratory failure*.

Treatment—*Atropine* to counteract muscarinic hyperstimulation; *pralidoxime (2-PAM)*

Carbamates

 Pyridostigmine, neostigmine, carbaryl

Mechanism of Toxicity—Inhibition of the enzyme acetylcholinesterase. Carbamates do not bind as strongly to the active site of the enzyme as organophosphorus compounds, and therefore are considered to be *"reversible" inhibitors* of acetylcholinesterase.

Toxic Effects—*SLUDE syndrome*, bronchoconstriction and increased bronchosecretions, muscular fasciculations, and, in severe cases, paralysis and death due to respiratory failure

Treatment—*Atropine* to counteract muscarinic hyperstimulation

Organochlorine Compounds

 Dichlorodiphenyltrichloroethane (DDT)

Mechanism of Toxicity—Interferes with Na^+ channels in excitable membranes, resulting in repetitive neuronal firing and excessive stimulation. Transport of Ca^{2+} is also inhibited.

Toxic Effects—CNS stimulation, tremors; convulsions and tetanic paralysis at higher doses

Treatment—Treatment is symptomatic; no agent specific treatment is available

Botanical Insecticides

These insecticides, including *nicotine*, *rotenone*, and *pyrethrum*, are derived from natural sources.

Nicotine

Mechanism of Toxicity—Stimulation of nicotinic cholinergic receptors

Toxic Effects—Stimulation is followed by desensitization, resulting in respiratory paralysis and death.

Treatment—Treatment is symptomatic; no agent-specific treatment is available

HERBICIDES

Bipyridyl Herbicides

 Paraquat (for crop dusting)

Mechanism of Toxicity—Excessive free radical oxidative damage

Toxic Effects—Gradual *accumulation in the lung* after exposure results in hemorrhagic pulmonary edema, alveolitis, and pulmonary fibrosis.

Treatment—Gastric lavage, adsorbents, and cathartics are used to prevent additional GI absorption; oxygen may aggravate pulmonary lesions, and should be used with caution

RODENTICIDES

Strychnine

Mechanism of Toxicity—Competitive antagonist at the glycine receptor, blocking the *inhibitory effects of glycine within the spinal cord* and resulting in diffuse excitatory effects

Toxic Effects—CNS excitation, causing diffuse muscle contraction, tetanic convulsions, and cessation of respiration due to diaphragmatic contraction

Treatment—Respiratory support and *diazepam* to ease convulsions. In severe cases, anesthesia or neuromuscular blockade may be needed to alleviate convulsions.

Warfarin

Mechanism of Toxicity—Oral anticoagulant that inhibits key factors in the clotting cascade

Toxic Effects—*Excessive bleeding*

Treatment—*Vitamin K* can overcome *warfarin*-dependent inhibition of clotting factor synthesis in approximately 24 hours; *fresh frozen plasma* can be used in cases of acute poisoning

HARDCORE

Organophosphorus compounds phosphorylate the active site of acetylcholinesterase. This bond is very stable and not easily reversible. The stability of this bond is further increased by the loss of an alkyl group, a process known as "aging." *Pralidoxime* can be administered to increase the rate of regeneration of acetylcholinesterase following exposure to an organophosphorus compound. However, *pralidoxime* will not work if the enzyme-inhibitor complex has "aged."

AIR POLLUTANTS

Many different air pollutants exist as the result of emission from industry, automobiles and other forms of transportation, power generation, and waste disposal. The primary organ affected by these compounds is *the lung*, although absorption and systemic distribution may also occur.

CARBON MONOXIDE (CO)

Mechanism of Toxicity—Combines with hemoglobin to form carboxyhemoglobin (COHb). COHb cannot carry oxygen, thus the *oxygen carrying capacity of the blood is reduced*. COHb also inhibits the dissociation of oxygen from oxyhemoglobin.

Toxic Effects—Toxic effects are *similar to hypoxia*. Specifically, the patient initially complains of a headache, which over time progresses to dimmed vision, vomiting, slowed respiration, and possibly death as the amount of COHb in the blood increases.

Treatment—Remove the source of CO, *administration of 100% oxygen*, monitor vital signs

SULFUR DIOXIDE (SO₂)

Generated by the *burning of fossil fuels.*

Mechanism of Toxicity—Following contact with moisture, forms the irritant *sulfurous acid*

Toxic Effects—Severe *irritation of the eyes, mucous membranes, and skin*; bronchoconstriction and possible *pulmonary edema* in severe cases

Treatment—Minimize irritation of respiratory tract and other tissues by limiting exposure, but no specific treatment is available

NITROGEN OXIDES

Mechanism of Toxicity—Irritation, especially of the deep lung

Toxic Effects—Irritation of the eyes and mucous membranes, dyspnea, chest pain, and pulmonary edema with *fibrotic destruction of terminal bronchioles*

Treatment—Maintenance of gas exchange and management of pulmonary edema, use of bronchodilators; no specific treatment is available

HARDCORE REVIEW – TOXICOLOGY

HARDCORE

Carbon monoxide makes blood *cherry red*.

TABLE 12-1	Common Therapeutic Drugs	
TOXIC AGENT	MAJOR CLINICAL EFFECTS	MAJOR ANTIDOTE (IF AVAILABLE)
Acetaminophen	Hepatic and renal tubular necrosis	N-acetylcysteine (NAC)
Ethanol	Vomiting, nausea, CNS depression	Withdrawal prophylaxis
Ethylene glycol	Acidosis and nephrotoxicity	Ethanol
Methanol	Severe acidosis, retinal damage	Ethanol
Aspirin	Uncompensated respiratory and metabolic acidosis	
Atropine	Anticholinergic effects	Physostigmine
Barbiturates	CNS, respiratory depression	
Benzodiazepines	CNS, respiratory depression	Flumazenil
Digitalis	Arrhythmias, nausea, vomiting, confusion, electrolyte abnormalities, visual disturbances	Digitalis-specific antibody Fab fragments
Fibrinolytic drugs	Hemorrhage	Aminocaproic acid
Heparin	Hemorrhage	Protamine sulfate
Opiates	CNS, respiratory depression	Naloxone or naltrexone

TABLE 12-2 Heavy Metals

Toxic Agent	Major Clinical Effects	Major Antidote (If Available)
Arsenic	Hyperpigmentation of skin, Mees lines, coma, ascending sensorimotor peripheral neuropathy	Dimercaprol (BAL) or succimer
Iron	Liver dysfunction, heart failure, skin pigmentation, and diabetes mellitus	Deferoxamine
Lead	Sleep disturbance, slowed reaction time, peripheral neuropathy and memory loss, anemia, nephrosclerosis, hypertension, lead lines on gingivae and epiphyses of long bones	Dimercaprol, EDTA
Mercury	Gingivostomatitis, pneumonitis, and pulmonary edema, neuropyschiatric disturbances	Dimercaprol (BAL) or succimer

TABLE 12-3 All Other Classes

Toxic Agent	Major Clinical Effects	Major Antidote (If Available)
Insecticides		
Organophosphorus compounds • Diisopropylflurophosphate • Nerve gases • Malathion	SLUDE syndrome, muscular fasciculations, respiratory failure	Atropine, 2-PAM
Carbamates • Pyridostigmine • Neostigmine • Carbaryl	SLUDE syndrome	Atropine
Organochlorine compound • DDT	CNS stimulation, tremors, followed by convulsions at higher doses	
Botanical insecticides • Nicotine	Respiratory paralysis and death	
• Rotenone	GI irritation and vomiting, respiratory depression, convulsions	
• Pyrethrum	Convulsions, tetanic paralysis, contact dermatitis	
Herbicides		
Bipyridyl herbicides Paraquat	Hemorrhagic pulmonary edema, alveolitis, pulmonary fibrosis	
Rodenticides		
Sodium fluoroacetate	Cardiac irregularities; cyanosis; convulsions; death resulting from ventricular fibrillation or respiratory failure	Acetate
Strychnine	Tetanic convulsions and cessation of respiration due to diaphragmatic contraction	
Warfarin	Hemorrhage	Vitamin K, fresh frozen plasma
Air Pollutants		
Carbon monoxide (CO)	Headache, dim vision, vomiting, slowed respiration, and death	100% oxygen
Sulfur oxides	Eye, mucous membrane, and skin irritation; bronchial constriction; pulmonary edema	
Nitrogen oxides	Cough, dypsnea, pulmonary edema	

TABLE 12-4	Specific Antidotes
ANTIDOTE	**TOXIC AGENT**
Acetate	Sodium fluoroacetate
Aminocaproic acid	Fibrinolytic drugs
Atropine	Organophosphorus compounds, carbamates
Deferoxamine	Iron
Digitalis-specific antibody Fab fragments	Digitalis
Dimercaprol (BAL)	Arsenic, mercury, gold, lead
EDTA	Lead
Ethanol	Ethylene glycol, methanol
Flumazenil	Benzodiazepines
Fresh frozen plasma	Warfarin
N-acetylcysteine (NAC)	Acetaminophen
Naloxone or naltrexone	Opiates
Oxygen (100%)	Carbon monoxide
2-PAM	Organophosphates
Physostigmine	Atropine
Protamine sulfate	Heparin
Succimer	Arsenic, mercury, gold, lead
Vitamin K	Warfarin

CHAPTER 13

Hardcore Board Concepts

Most of the pharmacology questions on your exam will be based on the fundamentals already presented in this book: indications, mechanism of action, and side effects. However, the board exam also expects you to know adverse properties of commonly used drugs, including drug allergies, teratogenic drugs, and cytochrome P450 drug inducers and inhibitors. You may be wondering why the board examiners care about such specific pharmacological properties. They want to be sure that next year, when you are on the wards, you will be aware of the important properties and major adverse effects associated with commonly used medications.

DRUGS ASSOCIATED WITH ADVERSE REACTIONS

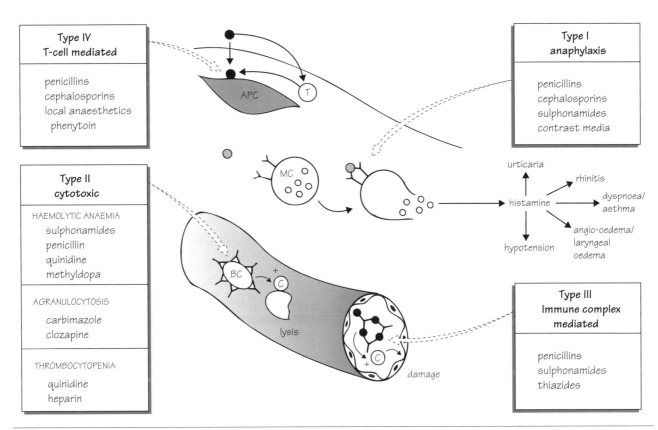

Figure 13-1 Adverse drug reactions. (Reprinted with permission from Neal MJ. Medical Pharmacology at a Glance. 4th ed. Oxford: Blackwell Publishing, 2002:96.)

Patients with *glucose-6-phosphate dehydrogenase (G6PD) deficiency may develop hemolytic anemia* if treated with *sulfonamide drugs, antimalarial agents (primaquine, hydrochloroquine),* or *dapsone.*

Sulfonamides

Allergic Mechanism—Drug metabolites attach to human proteins inducing an immune response.

Commonly Used Drugs Containing Sulfa

Refer to Table 13-1.

TABLE 13-1	Commonly Used Drugs Containing Sulfa		
ANTIBIOTICS	**DIURETICS**	**SULFONYLUREAS**	**OTHER**
Sulfamethoxazole	Furosemide	Clorpropamide	Acetazolamide
Sulfadiazine	Hydrochlorothiazide	Tolbutamide	
Sulfisoxazole	Indapamide	Tolazamide	
Sulfathiazole	Methyclothiazide	Glipizide	
Sulfacetamide	Chlorothiazide	Glyburide	

About 15% of people allergic to the *penicillins* will also be allergic to the *cephalosporins* (*cross-sensitivity*).

Beta-Lactamase Inhibitors

The penicillin allergy.

Allergic Mechanism—Drug metabolites react with endogenous proteins by acting as **haptens**, inducing an immune response (Table 13-2).

TABLE 13-2	Beta-Lactamase Inhibitors Associated with Penicillin Allergies			
PENICILLINS	**FIRST-GENERATION CEPHALOSPORINS**	**SECOND-GENERATION CEPHALOSPORINS**	**THIRD-GENERATION CEPHALOSPORINS**	**FOURTH-GENERATION CEPHALOSPORINS**
Penicillin G and V	Cefazolin	Cefaclor	Cefotaxime	Cefepime
Methicillin	Cephalexin	Cefoxitin	Ceftazidime	
Nafcillin		Cefuroxime	Ceftriaxone	
Ampicillin		Cefotetan	Cefixime	
Amoxicillin		Cefmetazole	Cefoperazone	
Ticarcillin				
Piperacillin				
Carbenicillin				

Other Common Drugs That May Cause Allergic Reactions

- *Latex*
- *Insulin*
- *Heparin*
- *Codeine*
- *Iodine*
- *Phenytoin*
- *Carbamazepine*
- *Valproic acid*

Heparin may cause thrombocytopenia and paradoxical thrombosis.

ENVIRONMENTAL ALLERGIES AND ANAPHYLAXIS

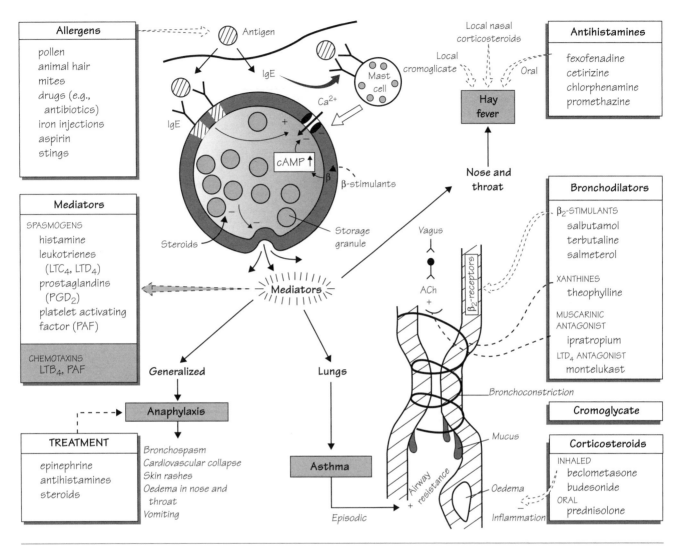

Figure 13-2 Asthma, hay fever, and anaphylaxis. Hyperreactive diseases are generally caused by the same basic principle. First, the allergen-specific immunoglobulin, IgE, attaches to mast cells after an inital exposure to an allergen. On subsequent exposure to the same antigen, mast cells degranulate, releasing mediators including histamine, leukotrienes, and prostaglandins, which trigger the allergy reaction. Anaphylaxis refers to a life-threatening response to an antigen that may result from the massive, general release of mast cell mediators. Treatment for these reactions is listed in the figure. (Reprinted with permission from Neal MJ. Medical Pharmacology at a Glance. 4th ed. Oxford: Blackwell Publishing, 2002:28.)

TERATOGENIC AND NONTERATOGENIC DRUGS

A **teratogen is an agent capable of causing malformations in a fetus**. Table 13-3 lists common teratogenic agents. Remember, the **fetus is most susceptible in the third to eighth week of pregnancy, during organogenesis**. Table 13-4 presents drugs that are safe for use during pregnancy. Table 13-5 lists safe alternatives for some commonly used teratogenic drugs. Table 13-6 lists some common drugs that are not safe for use during breastfeeding.

TABLE 13-3 Teratogenic Substances

Drug	Effect on Fetus
Ethanol—liquor	Congenital cardiac/CNS/limb anomalies, intrauterine growth retardation (IUGR), developmental delay, attention deficit, autism
Aspirin	Neonatal bleeding, prolonged gestation
ACE inhibitors—captopril, enalapril	Renal failure, oligohydramnios (*not enough amniotic fluid*)
Carbamazepine	Spina bifida/neural tube defects
Carbon monoxide	Cerebral atrophy, microcephaly
Chloroquine	Deafness
Chloramphenicol	Gray baby syndrome
Cigarette smoking	Low birth weight for gestational age
Ciprofloxacin	Problems with connective tissue development
Cocaine	Microcephaly, low birth weight (LBW), IUGR, behavioral disturbances
Corticosteroids (*systemic*)	LBW, premature delivery
Danazol	Virilization
Diethylstilbestrol (DES)	Vaginal clear cell adenocarcinoma when child is in adolescence
Ergotamines	Fetal growth retardation, miscarriage
Ibuprofen	Oligohydramnios
Imipramine	Limb defects and neonatal withdrawal syndrome
Iodide	Goiter
Isotretinoin	Face-ear anomalies, heart disease
Lithium	Ebstein's anomaly, macrosomia (if taken in the first trimester)
Penicillamine	Cutis laxa syndrome (*mutation in the elastin gene causing skin that is both lax and inelastic*)
Phenytoin	IUGR, neuroblastoma, bleeding (vitamin K deficiency)
Quinine	Thrombocytopenia, deafness
Streptomycin	Deafness
Sulfonamides	Kernicterus at low levels of serum bilirubin, hemolysis with G6PD deficiency
Sulfonylureas (*oral antidiabetics*)	Fetal hypoglycemia, ocular and bone abnormalities
Tetracyclines—tetracycline, doxycycline, minocycline	Pigmentation of teeth, retarded skeletal growth, limb malformations, cataracts, hypoplasia of enamel
Thalidomide	Deafness, phocomelia (*defective development of arms/legs so that the hands and feet are attached close to the body, resembling the flippers of a seal*)
Valproate	Spina bifida/neural tube defects
Vitamin D	Supravalvular aortic stenosis, hypercalcemia
Warfarin	Congenital malformations including nasal hypoplasia, optic atrophy, microcephaly, mental retardation

TABLE 13-4 Drugs That Can Be Used Safely During Pregnancy

CONDITION	SAFE MEDICATIONS
Allergies/rhinitis	Diphenhydramine, astemizole, cromolyn
Antibiotics	Azithromycin, cephalosporins, penicillins, nystatin
Bipolar affective disorder	Chlorpromazine, haloperidol
Constipation	Lactulose, docusate, mineral oil
Cough	Diphenhydramine, codeine, dextromethorphan
Depression	Tricyclics (TCAs), fluoxetine
Diabetes	Insulin
Hypertension	Labetalol, methyldopa
Migraine	Acetaminophen, codeine, TCAs/beta-blockers for prophylaxis
Nausea	Chlorpromazine, diphenhydramine
Neuromuscular blocking agents	Succinylcholine
Peptic ulcer	Antacids, sucralfate, bismuth, ranitidine
Pruritus	Hydroxyzine, diphenhydramine
Seizures	Phenobarbital
Thrombophlebitis	Heparin

TABLE 13-5 Alternative Drugs for Use During Pregnancy

INSTEAD OF THESE DRUGS . . .	. . . USE THESE
Ciprofloxacin or doxycycline	Azithromycin
Carbamazepine or phenytoin	Phenobarbital
Warfarin or aspirin	Heparin
ACE inhibitor	Methyldopa or labetalol
Sulfonylureas	Insulin
Sumatriptan or ibuprofen	Acetaminophen

TABLE 13-6 Drugs That Are Not Safe for Use While Breastfeeding

Amphetamines
Bromocriptine
Cimetidine
Chloramphenicol
Cocaine
Cyclophosphamide
Cyclosporine
DES
Doxorubicin
Ergot alkaloids
Heroin
Immunosuppressants
Iodides
Lithium
Methimazole
Nicotine
Phencyclidine
Tetracycline
Thiouracil

CYTOCHROME P-450 DRUG INDUCERS AND INHIBITORS

Remember that drug metabolic reactions in the liver are catalyzed by isoforms of the *cytochrome P-450 system*. Agents that interact with this system can cause an up-regulation of specific P-450 isozymes, resulting in a more rapid clearance and lower concentration of other drugs. Drugs with this side effect are known as cytochrome P-450 *inducers*. Other agents inhibit the P-450 system and can slow the metabolism of drugs that are metabolized by this system, thereby raising their plasma concentrations. Drugs with this side effect are known as cytochrome P-450 *inhibitors*. A large number of drugs interact with the P-450 system; Table 13-7 lists some of the most common agents that show up on board exams.

TABLE 13-7	Inducers of the Cytochrome P-450 Enzyme			
RIFAMYCINS	CORTICOSTEROIDS	ANTICONVULSANTS	ORAL HYPOGLYCEMIC AGENTS	OTHER
Rifabutin	Dexamethasone	Phenobarbital	Troglitazone	Ethanol
Rifampin	Prednisone	Phenytoin	Pioglitazone	Griseofulvin
		Carbamazepine		Modafinil
				Omeprazol
				INH

The most common and testable **inducers** can be remembered with the mnemonic shown in Figure 13-3 and Table 13-8.

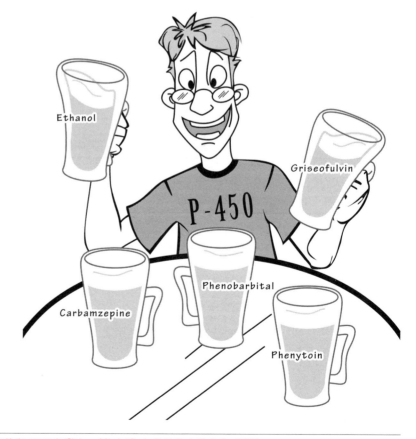

INDUCERS OF CYTOCHROME P-450

Pitchers Of Alcohol Can Be Pretty Good At Inducing P-450

Pitchers - phenobarbital
of **A**lcohol - Ethanol
Can - Carbamzepine
be **P**retty - Phenytoin
Good - Griseofulvin
at **I**nducing **P-450**

Figure 13-3 Remember the most common inducers of cytochrome P-450 with the mnemonic "Pitchers of Alcohol Can be Pretty Good at **i**nducing P450."

TABLE 13-8 Inhibitors of the Cytochrome P-450 Enzyme

HISTAMINE BLOCKERS	ANTIFUNGAL	ANTIBIOTICS	CARDIOVASCULAR	PROTEASE INHIBITORS	OTHER
Cimetidine	Ketoconazole	Erythromycin	Amiodarone	Indinavir	Lovastatin
Ranitidine	Itraconazole	Clarithromycin	Verapamil	Nelfinavir	Fluoxetine
Diphenhydramine	Fluconazole	Chloramphenicol	Quinidine		Gemfibrozil
Hydroxyzine		Isoniazid	Lovastatin		Zafirlukast
		Trimethoprim			Celecoxib
		Sulfamethoxazole			Probenecid
		Ciprofloxacin			Indomethacin

The most common and testable **inhibitors** can be remembered with the mnemonic shown in Figure 13-4.

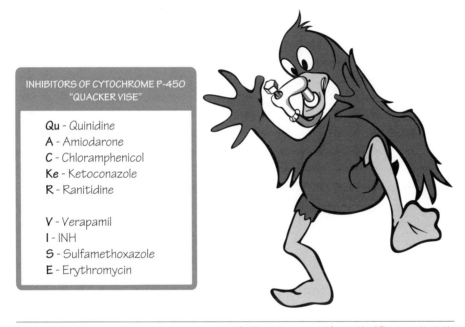

INHIBITORS OF CYTOCHROME P-450
"QUACKER VISE"

Qu - Quinidine
A - Amiodarone
C - Chloramphenicol
Ke - Ketoconazole
R - Ranitidine

V - Verapamil
I - INH
S - Sulfamethoxazole
E - Erythromycin

Figure 13-4 Remember the most common inhibitors of cytochrome P-450 with the mnemonic "Quacker Vise." The vise on this duck's bill is *inhibiting* it from quacking!

CHAPTER 14

Hardcore Figures and Graphs

In addition to the standard board test question, the USMLE Step 1 will test your thought process and interpretation of scientific data with questions that require you to interpret figures and graphs that can be intimidating and complex. Despite their appearance, most of these questions are readily answerable, and answering them correctly can really help your final score. Although you will see these questions on all board topics, the pharmacology section tends to use these questions more than most other areas. Below we will give you the tools to take on these questions fearlessly and ultimately improve your final score.

Often, these questions will use graphs with multiple colors, bars, and lines. When you see a graph, remember the following:

1. Do not panic, become agitated, or press the "next question" box.

2. Take a deep breath and read the question without paying any attention to the graph or figure.

3. You will find that often these questions ask you to identify a basic concept typically involving one of the following:
   a. Pharmacokinetics
   b. Pharmacology of the autonomic nervous system
   c. Side effect or actions of a single drug or one drug compared to another

4. Attempt to answer the question in your head before even looking at the graph. Sometimes the question will be formatted so that you won't be able to do this. Don't worry, if you know what concept they are testing, you will be fine.

5. Now take a look at the graph. First look at the format of the graph. What type of graph is it? What are the X- and Y-axes? What are the units of measurement?

6. If you have spent more than 15–20 seconds reading the initial question and you do not understand what it is asking, or if you are looking at the graph and are unfamiliar with the formatting or axes, click one of the answers, mark this question, and come back after you have answered the rest of the questions in this section.

Try these representative questions:

QUESTION #1

First, look at the question without paying any attention to the graph:

The changes in heart rate and bronchiole smooth muscle tension are illustrated above (in the graph) following pretreatment with either albuterol or metoprolol and the addition of drug X. The illustration shows the effect of drug X, but not the effect of either pretreatment. What is drug X?

What concept is this question asking you to identify?

Albuterol and metoprolol both act on β-adrenergic receptors in the autonomic nervous system, but their primary actions are on different receptor subtypes, accounting for differences in side effects. There are two major subtypes of β-adrenergic receptors: β_1 *and* β_2. β_1 receptors are found primarily in the heart and act to increase heart rate and contractility. β_2 receptors are found chiefly in smooth muscle cells in the blood vessels and bronchioles and, when stimulated, cause smooth muscle relaxation and ultimately vasodilation and bronchodilation.

Metoprolol is a β_1 blocker, used to treat hypertension. Albuterol is a β_2 agonist, used to treat asthma. Even though we know nothing about drug X, we know the effects of albuterol and metoprolol on heart rate and smooth muscle tone. Metoprolol, a β_1 selective adrenergic receptor antagonist, produces a decrease in heart rate due to the blockade of the action of endogenous catecholamines. Metoprolol would not be expected to have much effect on bronchiolar smooth muscle, since it acts selectively on β_1-adrenergic receptors and not β_2-adrenergic receptors. Albuterol, a β_2 selective adrenergic receptor agonist, should dilate smooth muscle, increasing

HARDCORE

- β_1-**adrenergic receptors**—Increase heart rate, increase myocardial contractility, increase renin release, and promote lipolysis.

- β_2-**adrenergic receptors**—Vasodilation, bronchodilation, increase glucagon release.

bronchiolar diameter, and would not be expected to have a large effect on heart rate, because it has a low affinity for β_1-adrenergic receptors. Without even looking at the graph, we can deduce that drug X will likely act on β-adrenergic receptors to some degree, since both albuterol and metoprolol act on β receptors.

Now let's take a look at the graph. *What type of graph is it? What are the axes? Do the bars represent an increase or decrease in the parameter being represented?*

This is a bar graph representing the effect of drug X following pretreatment with either albuterol or metoprolol, on heart rate and bronchiolar smooth muscle tone. Notice that the Y-axis differs in each graph. The baseline starts at "0" for both heart rate and bronchiolar smooth muscle tension. In the upper graph, the change in heart rate from baseline moves in the positive direction, indicating an increase in heart rate. This is consistent with the action of a β_1-adrenergic receptor agonist, which acts on the heart to increase heart rate. In contrast, in the lower graph, the bronchiolar smooth muscle tension bars move in the negative direction, indicating a decrease in bronchiolar smooth muscle tension, or an increase in bronchiole diameter. This effect is consistent with the action of a β_2-adrenergic receptor agonist.

We see that drug X increases heart rate when combined with albuterol, as illustrated by the increase in the height of the bar in the upper half of the graph. Since albuterol is a β_2 selective agonist and does not act on the heart, we know that drug X must have some intrinsic β_1 agonist activity to account for the increase in heart rate. Additionally, the combination of drug X and albuterol produces marked bronchiolar dilation. Therefore, we can be pretty sure that, in addition to β_1 agonist activity, drug X also has some degree of activity at β_2-adrenergic receptors. In the metoprolol-pretreated group, heart rate remains near baseline when drug X is added, which is expected because of metoprolol's β_1-adrenergic receptor blocking action. However, drug X causes a decrease in bronchiolar smooth muscle tension when combined with metoprolol. Since metoprolol is a selective β_1-adrenergic receptor antagonist that does not act on β_2 receptors, it suggests that drug X possesses some β_2-adrenergic receptor activity, resulting in bronchiolar dilation. So, before we even look at the answer list, we know that ***drug X is a β_1 and β_2 agonist***.

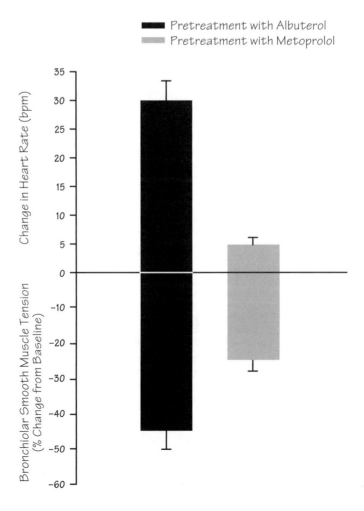

Figure 14-1

The rest of the question:

What is drug X?
A. Edrophonium
B. Phentolamine
C. Epinephrine
D. Norepinephrine
E. Nadolol

Of the possible answer choices, only *epinephrine* **(C)** is a **nonselective β agonist**. Let's go through the other choices:

A. The anticholinesterase agent *edrophonium* would be expected to slow the heart rate and increase bronchiole smooth muscle tension, since it potentiates the effects of acetylcholine. Drug X increases heart rate and diminishes bronchiole smooth muscle tone, so we know that *edrophonium* is not drug X.

B. *Phentolamine* is a nonselective α-adrenergic receptor antagonist that can induce reflex tachycardia, but does not have any significant influence on β_2 receptors or bronchiole smooth muscle tension. Therefore, we can safely rule out *phentolamine*.

D. *Norepinephrine* acts as an agonist primarily at α_1-, α_2-, and β_1-adrenergic receptors, and, therefore, would have minimal β_2-mediated smooth muscle dilating effects seen with drug X.

E. *Nadolol* is a nonselective β-adrenergic receptor blocker. Drug X is a nonselective β-receptor agonist that can increase heart rate via β_1 receptor activation and decrease bronchiolar smooth muscle tension via action at β_2-adrenergic receptors, so we know drug X is not *nadolol*.

QUESTION #2

First, the question:

The in vivo metabolism of cyclosporine is illustrated following the addition of increasing doses of drug Y (0.1 mg, 0.3 mg, and 1.0 mg) to the patient. What is drug Y?

What concept is this question asking you to identify?

This question is asking about drug metabolism, a ***pharmacokinetic property***. Before going any further, what do we know about drug metabolism? We know the liver is the major site for drug metabolism and most drugs that undergo metabolic transformation follow a first-order kinetic reaction causing a *constant fraction of the drug to be metabolized per unit time*. This question is inquiring about the influence of an unknown drug (Y) on the metabolism of cyclosporine. We should be aware that this question is asking us to identify a drug that may interfere with the metabolism of cyclosporine. *How is cyclosporin metabolized?*

Now let's look at the graph. *What type of graph is it and what are the axes? Do the bars represent an increase or decrease in the metabolism of cyclosporine?*

On this bar graph, the Y-axis represents the metabolism of cyclosporine in μg/min. Its baseline starts at "0," and the bars move in the positive direction, indicating the rate at which the cyclosporine is metabolized. This rate decreases as drug Y is added in increasing doses, suggesting that drug Y interferes with the metabolism of cyclosporine in some way. Let's look at the possible answers.

HARDCORE

Drugs metabolized in the liver are catalyzed by isoforms of the cytochrome P-450 system. Certain drugs influence the concentration of these enzymes and change the rate of metabolism of other drugs.

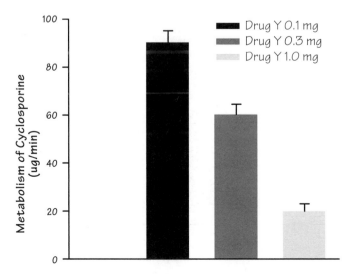

Figure 14-2

Key inhibitors of the cytochrome P-450 system: *Quinidine, amiodarone, cimetidine, ketoconazole, ranitidine, verapamil, isoniazid, ciprofloxacin,* and *erythromycin.*

Key inducers of the cytochrome P-450 system: *Ethanol, carbamazepine, rifampin, phenobarbital, phenytoin,* and *griseofulvin.*

What is drug Y?

A. **Griseofulvin**
B. **Erythromycin**
C. **Penicillin**
D. **Tetracycline**
E. **Ticarcillin**

Of the possible answer choices, only **erythromycin** (B), which inhibits the P-450 system, influencing the metabolism of other drugs, would interfere with the metabolism of cyclosporin, and therefore is drug Y. Griseofulvin induces the P-450 system, and would be expected to enhance the metabolism of cyclosporin. The other answer choices do not affect the metabolism of cyclosporin, because they do not significantly alter the P450 system, and therefore would not be expected to influence the metabolism of cyclosporine.

QUESTION #3

First the question:

Below is a graph that shows the percent survival over time for patients enrolled in a clinical trial of drug K. Circles indicate that a subject has been censored (dropped from the study) at the indicated time. The subjects were censored for various health reasons that caused them to be too ill to continue on the study protocol. How are the data collected on drug K likely to be affected by the censored subjects in this study?

What type of graph is this, and what are the axes? The graph is a **survival curve**, and is commonly used to represent the results of a clinical trial. The Y-axis represents the percent of subjects still alive at the time point indicated on the X-axis. Each open circle on the graph represents a subject that has been dropped from the study (censored) due to illness. Each downward jump in the curve represents the death of one or more patients in the study. Note that a "survival" curve does not have to use death as an endpoint. Other endpoints, such as recovery from a particular surgery, may be encountered.

Now let's look at the possible answers:

A. **The censored subjects will not affect the survival curve.**
B. **The data on the remaining subjects will overestimate the survival of the entire population.**
C. **The data on the remaining subjects will underestimate the survival of the entire population.**
D. **The data on the remaining subjects will overestimate the survival of the entire population at points fewer than 15 months, and will underestimate the survival of the entire population for points greater than 15 months.**

Since the subjects who were censored were sicker than those who remained in the study, it is likely that the censored subjects will die before the uncensored subjects. Therefore, the subjects remaining in the study will die later than the average of the entire population (*censored + uncensored subjects*), resulting in an overestimation of the survival of the population by the graph.

The correct answer is (B).

Note that this question tests your knowledge of survival curves, while not actually requiring you to read any values from the graph that is given. If you read the question and were familiar with survival curves, you may not have needed to look at the graph at all!

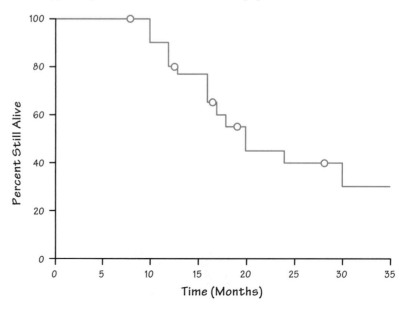

Figure 14-3

QUESTION #4

First the question:

The following table lists information about four different drugs. A loading dose of 20 mg of each drug was given. Based on the loading dose and the information provided in the table, which of the drugs (A–D) has the largest volume of distribution?

After reading the question, we know that the major concept is *volume of distribution* (V_D), and we can't answer the question without some of the information that is given in the table. Recall from the pharmacokinetics review that volume of distribution refers to the *relationship between the dose of a drug given to the measured plasma concentration of the drug*. This can be calculated by:

$$V_D = \text{Loading dose}/C_o$$

Where V_D is the apparent volume of distribution, and C_o is the initial concentration of the drug measured in the plasma following distribution of the drug.

Now let's look at the table that's given:

TABLE 14-1	Question # 4			
DRUG	MOLECULAR WEIGHT (G/MOL)	PLASMA CONCENTRATION FOLLOWING DISTRIBUTION (MG/ML)	% BOUND BY PLASMA PROTEINS	ELIMINATION CLEARANCE (ML/HR)
A	123	0.70	17	11
B	27	1.10	7	24
C	589	0.04	4	2
D	212	4.35	1	110

And now let's look at the possible choices:

A. Drug A
B. Drug B
C. Drug C
D. Drug D

Using the formula and the information given about loading dose and the concentration of each drug in the plasma, the V_D for each drug can be calculated. However, it is not necessary to actually calculate the V_D for each drug, since the question is not asking for the actual value. All that is needed is to determine which drug has the largest V_D. Since the loading dose of each drug is identical (20 mg), the V_D for each drug is inversely proportional to the C_o. Drug C has the smallest C_o, and, thus, the largest V_D.

The correct answer is C.

Now try a couple of questions on your own:

QUESTION #5

The figure below represents a diagram of the neurogenic signaling cascade for the constriction of vascular smooth muscle. When infused into this neurovascular system, drug X has no influence on the degree or frequency of vascular smooth muscle constriction. Which of the following drugs is most likely to be drug X?

A. Phenylephrine
B. Methoxamine
C. Clonidine
D. Isoproterenol

The correct answer is D. Isoproterenol is a β-adrenergic receptor agonist and will not stimulate the α-adrenergic receptors represented in the diagram. Phenylephrine and methoxamine are both α_1-adrenergic agonists, and will result in constriction of vascular smooth muscle. Clonidine is an α_2-adrenergic agonist and will result in decreased norepinephrine (NE) release and relaxation of vascular smooth muscle.

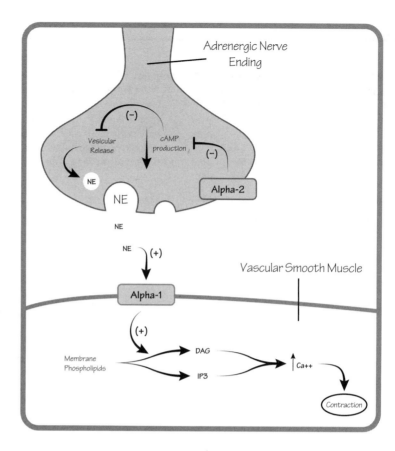

Figure 14-4

QUESTION #6

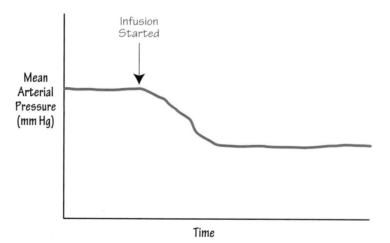

Figure 14-5

An infusion of which of the following drugs will produce the observed effect on mean arterial pressure?

A. Atropine
B. Angiotensin II
C. Carbachol
D. Phenylephrine

The correct answer is **C.** Only an infusion of carbachol, a muscarinic receptor agonist, will produce a drop in blood pressure. An infusion of either angiotensin II or phenylephrine would result in an increase in mean arterial pressure. An infusion of atropine would not greatly change mean arterial pressure, since there is very little endogenous cholinergic tone in the vascular system.

QUESTION #7

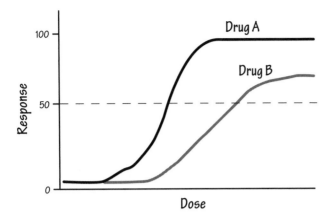

Figure 14-6

Which of the following statements about drugs A and B is correct?

A. Drug A is less potent than drug B.
B. Drug A is more potent and more efficacious than drug B.
C. Drug B is less potent, but equally as efficacious as drug A.
D. Drug A is less potent, but equally as efficacious as drug B.
E. Drug B is more potent, but less efficacious than drug A.
F. Drugs A and B have equal potency and efficacy.

The correct answer is B. Remember efficacy can be determined by identifying the maximum response that a drug can produce, regardless of the dose at which that response occurs. By looking at the graph, it can be seen that drug A is more efficacious than drug B since it produces a greater maximal response. This eliminates choices C, D, and F. Potency can de determined from the graph by looking at the EC_{50} for each drug. The EC_{50} is the dose of drug at which a half-maximal response is produced. More potent drugs have lower EC_{50} values, because less of the drug is necessary to produce the desired response. The graph demonstrates that drug A is more potent, since the dose at which it produces a half-maximal response is less than that of drug B. This eliminates choices A and E, leaving only choice B. The dashed line going across the graph at 50 has no meaning in the problem, and is included only as a distraction.

QUESTION #8

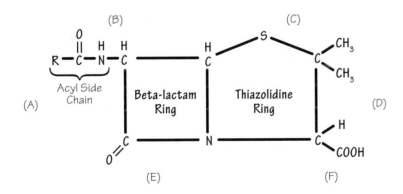

Figure 14-7

At which part of the penicillin molecule do β-lactamases act?

A.
B.
C.
D.
E.
F.

The correct answer is E. β-lactamase enzymes render penicillins, and other β-lactam antibiotics, inactive by irreversibly cleaving the lactam ring through irreversible hydroxylation of the amide bond (E). β-lactamases are a common resistance mechanism among gram-positive and gram-negative organisms, both aerobic and anaerobic. β-lactamases do not alter the structure at any other site.

QUESTION #9

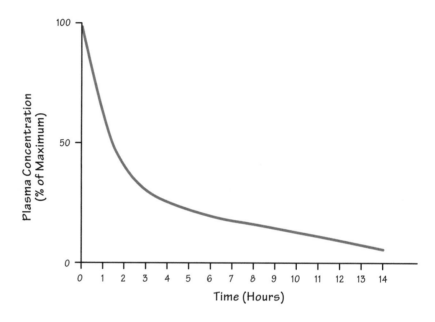

Figure 14-8

Above is a graph showing the plasma concentration of drug X versus time. Drug X was administered at time = 0. Which of the following statements regarding drug X is correct?

A. The half-life of drug X is approximately 3 hours.
B. Drug X was most likely given orally.
C. If drug X is infused at a constant rate intravenously, it will reach steady state after 4–5 half-lives.
D. Drug X is most likely not lipophilic.
E. The bioavailability of drug X cannot be calculated from the above graph.

The correct answer is C. Choice (C) is the correct answer because any drug infused at a constant rate intravenously will reach steady state after 4–5 half-lives. The half-life is about 1 hour; therefore choice (A) is incorrect. There is no distribution phase on the curve suggesting that the drug was given intravenously; therefore choice (B) is not correct. Nothing about the lipophilic properties of drug X can be determined from the above graph, therefore choice (D) is incorrect. The bioavailability of drug X is the area under the concentration versus time curve for the given route of administration, divided by the area under the concentration versus time curve for the same drug given intravenously. In this case, drug X was given intravenously, making the bioavailability equal to 1 ($AUC_{iv}/AUC_{iv} = 1$); thus, choice (E) is not correct.

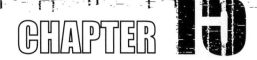

CHAPTER 15

Step 1 Practice Questions and Answers

1. A 43-year-old patient with a medical history of HIV, diabetes, and peripheral vascular disease is admitted into the hospital for severe dehydration. After several days of intravenous hydration, the patient develops oral thrush and is given nystatin to swish and swallow. Nystatin acts by:
   A. Binding ergosterol and forming transmembrane pores
   B. Blocking fungal ergosterol synthesis
   C. Interfering with fungal microtubule function to disrupt mitosis
   D. Binding ergosterol and disrupting fungal membranes

2. A 3-year-old child arrives in the emergency room after developing acute lead toxicity. An antidote for this crisis is:
   A. Penicillamine
   B. Succimer
   C. Deferoxamine
   D. Thiosulfate

3. A 37-year-old patient with a history of type I diabetes, asthma, and hypertension arrives at your clinic complaining of severe pain, redness, and swelling in his first metatarsal. The diagnosis of acute gouty arthritis is made and the patient is started on medication. Which medication is used for an acute attack of gout?
   A. Probenecid
   B. Allopurinol
   C. Colchicine
   D. Sulfinpyrazone

4. A 26-year-old patient with chronic asthma has required increasing amounts of asthma medications over the past 2 weeks due to a respiratory virus. She arrives in your office wheezing heavily and complaining of worsening shortness of breath that is only moderately relieved with albuterol. You decide to start a short course of beclomethasone. What is the mechanism of action of this drug?
   A. It blocks the synthesis of lipoxygenase
   B. It inhibits the enzyme phospholipase-A_2
   C. It competitively blocks muscarinic receptors
   D. It inhibits the enzyme phosphodiesterase

5. While volunteering in a free clinic, you meet a 23-year-old pregnant woman who recently emigrated from West Africa. She informs you that before she emigrated, she finished a course of chloramphenicol for a respiratory infection during an early period of her pregnancy. After hearing this, you become concerned for her unborn child. What fetal complication can this medication cause?
   A. Kernicterus
   B. Tooth staining
   C. Thrombocytopenia
   D. Gray baby syndrome

6. A 38-year-old African-American patient with a past medical history of sickle cell trait, glucose 6-phosphate dehydrogenase (G6PD) deficiency, type II diabetes, and gout arrives at the emergency department after developing jaundice, pallor, dark urine, and abdominal pain. The patient claims these symptoms began after he started taking a new medication. What medication did this patient most likely recently start?
   A. Glipizide
   B. Indomethacin
   C. Neomycin
   D. Aztreonam

7. Aminoglycosides act as protein synthesis inhibitors. On which ribosomal subunit do these drugs act?
   A. 30S
   B. 50S
   C. 70S
   D. 80S

8. A 58-year-old patient suffering from chronic rheumatoid arthritis has been taking NSAIDs for a number of years to control inflammation and pain. Over the past few months, the patient developed a gastroduodenal ulcer that required hospitalization after an episode of acute hypotension and melena. Due to the complications of chronic NSAID use, the patient is recently started on methotrexate. On which phase of the cell cycle does methotrexate act?
   A. M phase
   B. S phase
   C. G2 phase
   D. Methotrexate is non-cell cycle specific

9. A 22-year-old patient is brought to the emergency room by her mother after developing confusion, intermittent convulsions, tachycardia, and arrhythmias. After questioning her mother, you learn that the patient has past medical history of type I diabetes, anemia, cycloplegia, and major depression disorder, and that the mother discovered an empty medicine bottle in the patient's bathroom. You suspect that the patient ingested toxic levels of this medication. What medication did the patient probably overdose on?
   A. Sertraline
   B. Thioridazine
   C. Phenelzine
   D. Trazodone
   E. Nefazadone
   F. Amitriptyline
   G. Erythropoietin
   H. Metformin
   I. Insulin

10. An elderly hypertensive gentleman with a long medical history comes to your office complaining of a chronic, nonproductive cough. While taking his history, you discover that he has had this cough for the past 6 months. He also reports some episodes of dizziness and night sweats, although these only occur approximately once per month. He tells you that his primary reason for coming to your office is that this cough causes him embarrassment in social situations. You suspect this cough may be a side effect of his medications. Which of his medications may be responsible for his complaint?
   A. Furosemide
   B. Nifedipine
   C. Lisinopril
   D. Losartan

11. A 67-year-old man arrives at the emergency department complaining of chest pain and shortness of breath. He reports a crushing, substernal pain that radiates to his left shoulder and jaw, which has not subsided for the past hour despite the administration of multiple sublingual nitroglycerin tablets. Immediately he is given oxygen, morphine for the pain, and an aspirin. His ECG is recorded and a series of blood tests are done, and the tests indicate that he is having a myocardial infarction. He is given the medication abciximab and taken directly to the cardiac catheterization lab. What is abciximab's mechanism of action within the cardiovascular system?
   A. It inhibits platelet adenosine uptake
   B. It inhibits ADP receptors on platelets
   C. It inhibits prostaglandin production
   D. It blocks the glycoprotein IIb/IIa receptor

12. A 5-year-old child arrives to the emergency room after her parents found her this morning in a comatose state. The child is quickly examined and transferred to the pediatric intensive care unit. Despite extensive medical support, she eventually passes away 5 days later from fulminant hepatitis and cerebral edema. What medication did this child most likely ingest prior to her hospitalization to cause her condition?
   A. Indomethacin
   B. Aspirin
   C. Ampicillin
   D. Chloramphenicol

13. The antibiotic imipenem acts to prevent both the elongation and the cross-linking of bacterial cell wall peptidoglycan by inhibiting bacterial peptidases and penicillin binding proteins. Which of the following is a serious side effect associated with the use of imipenem?
    A. Seizures
    B. Thrombocytopenia
    C. Pseudomembranous colitis
    D. Ototoxicity

14. A 68-year-old patient with a history of Wolff-Parkinson-White syndrome presents with shortness of breath and bilateral pitting lower leg edema. Which of the following cardio-vascular medications is contraindicated in this patient?
    A. Warfarin
    B. Hydralazine
    C. Digoxin
    D. Captopril

15. A 44-year-old patient with a history of gastroesophageal reflux disease asks her physician why omeprazol is taken only once per day. Which of the following best explains why omeprazol is taken only once per day?
    A. It binds to the H^+/K^+-ATPase enzyme in parietal cells
    B. It irreversibly inhibits the proton pump
    C. It is hepatically cleared
    D. It is administered orally

16. A 56-year-old patient is hospitalized following a serious episode of pneumonia. While hospitalized, the on-call physician is called to the patient's room after the nurse found the patient short of breath and complaining of "a racing heart." The patient's ECG indicates supraventricular tachycardia (SVT). The doctor considers the use of either propranolol or verapamil to slow the patient's heart rate. What mechanism enables these drugs to alleviate supraventricular tachycardia?
    A. Prolongation of the QT interval
    B. Slowing of atrioventricular node conduction velocity
    C. Prolongation of the effective refractory period
    D. Diminution of heart contractility

17. A 33-year-old patient with a past medical history of asthma and juvenile rheumatoid arthritis visits his physician after several days of serious diarrhea of unknown origin and is administered loperamide. What is loperamide's mechanism of action?
    A. Adsorbs intestinal toxins and microorganisms
    B. Prostaglandin E_1 analog
    C. Activates opioid receptors in the enteric nervous system
    D. Blocks opioid receptors in the enteric nervous system

18. A 39-year-old female is diagnosed with bacterial vaginosis and is prescribed metronidazole. The next evening during dinner, the patient experiences an uncomfortable flushing sensation along with nausea, chest palpitations and pain, vertigo, and eventually hypotension and goes to the emergency room. Which of the following did the physician forget to warn his patient about ingesting while taking metronidazole?
    A. Cheese
    B. Milk
    C. Aspirin
    D. Alcohol

19. A 28-year-old female, who is taking warfarin because of a history of deep vein thrombosis, has recently discovered she is pregnant. Which medication should she take for this medical condition during her pregnancy?
    A. Urokinase
    B. Warfarin
    C. Heparin
    D. She should not take any medications during her pregnancy

20. A patient has been taking warfarin for chronic atrial fibrillation. During routine lab screening, his blood coagulation time is found to be abnormally increased. He reports that several days ago he started taking new medication. Which medication did he most likely recently start taking?
    A. Amiodarone
    B. Griseofulvin

C. Phenobarbital
D. Carbamazepine

21. A woman you have been seeing as a patient for a number of years comes to your clinic 2 weeks after being prescribed a new medication. She complains of generalized gastrointestinal distress including anorexia, mild nausea, and flatulence, along with pruritus. The results of her blood work show her liver enzymes to be significantly elevated. Which drug is most likely responsible for this elevation?
A. Ciprofloxacin
B. Tetracycline
C. Procainamide
D. Hydrochlorothiazide
E. Insulin
F. Glipizide
G. Losartan
H. Simvastatin
I. Captopril

22. A 6-year-old female complaining of painful burning with urination is brought to the emergency room by her mother. No abnormal findings were discovered following an extensive history and physical. She is diagnosed with a urinary tract infection and prescribed a medication. Which of the following medications is contraindicated in this patient?
A. Ceftriaxone
B. Trimethoprim/sulfamethoxazole
C. Aztreonam
D. Ciprofloxacin

23. A company has synthesized a β-lactam containing antibiotic. Which site on this molecule would be of concern to the company, given the known mechanism(s) of resistance present in bacteria?
A. Site A
B. Site B
C. Site C
D. Site D
E. Site E

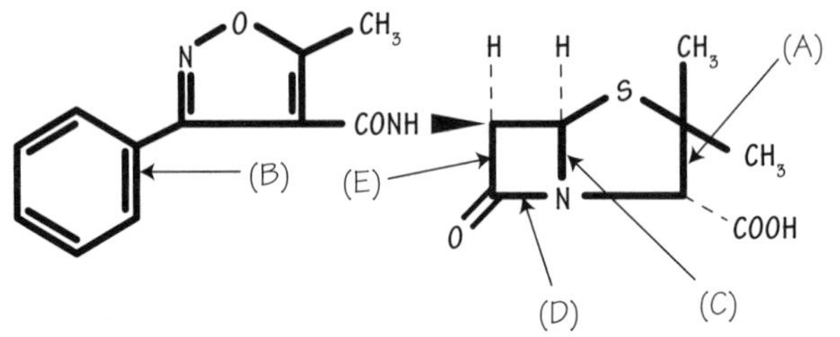

Figure 15-1 Question # 23

24. 5 mg of Drug Y are given intravenously to a patient. The concentration measured in the blood immediately after administration is 1 mg/L. You are told that the elimination of drug Y is first-order and that its clearance is 100 ml/hour. Approximately how long will it take for the concentration of drug Y in the blood to drop to 0.25 mg/L?
A. 34.5 hours
B. 17.25 hours
C. 69 hours
D. 72 hours

25. Carbachol eye drops produce miosis due to the ability of carbachol to simulate muscarinic receptors on the pupillary sphincter muscle, resulting in its contraction. Theoretically, an agent that produces mydriasis could antagonize the effect of carbachol. Which of the following is an example of a compound that would be considered a physiologic antagonist to carbachol's miotic effect?
A. A compound that produces mydriasis by stimulating α-adrenergic receptors on the radial muscles of the iris
B. A compound that produces mydriasis by blocking the muscarinic receptors to which carbachol binds on the pupillary sphincter
C. A compound that binds to and inactivates carbachol before it can stimulate its receptor
D. A compound that prevents the absorption of carbachol through the surface of the eye

1. D

Nystatin is a superficial antifungal agent clinically used for cutaneous or mucocutaneous (oral/vaginal) candidiasis infections. Nystatin acts by binding ergosterol and disrupting fungal cell membranes, resulting in altered membrane permeability and ultimately cell lysis. Amphotericin B binds to ergosterol and forms transmembrane pores (A). Terbinafine blocks ergosterol synthesis by inhibiting squalene epoxidase (B). Griseofulvin inhibits fungal microtubule function (C).

2. B

Patients presenting with potential acute lead toxicity should be treated with one of the following chelating agents: succimer, dimercaprol, or calcium disodium EDTA ($CaNa_2EDTA$). Penicillamine is a chelator used for copper, arsenic, and gold toxicity (A). Deferoxamine is used for iron toxicity (C). Thiosulfate is used for cyanide toxicity (D).

3. C

Gout is a metabolic disorder characterized by the deposition of urate crystals in joint spaces, resulting in inflammatory arthritis, tenosynovitis, and tophi accumulation. Acute attacks of gouty arthritis are readily responsive to colchicine and NSAIDs (e.g., aspirin or indomethacin), which limit granulocyte mobility and inflammation, respectively. The antihyperuricemic agents probenecid (A), allopurinol (B), and sulfinpyrazone (D) have limited use for acute attacks, because these agents do not limit the movement of immune cells or the inflammatory reaction that are characteristic of acute gouty attacks. Rather, these agents are used prophylactically to reduce the serum urate concentration, either by enhancing renal excretion of uric acid (uricosuric agents such as probenecid and sulfinpyrazone) or by decreasing uric acid synthesis (xanthine oxidase inhibitors such as allopurinol).

4. B

Beclomethasone is a corticosteroid that acts by inhibiting the enzyme phospholipase-A_2. Inhibiting phospholipase-A_2 decreases the production of prostaglandins and leukotrienes, ultimately suppressing the inflammatory response associated with asthma. Zileuton prevents leukotriene synthesis by blocking the synthesis of the enzyme lipoxygenase (A). Ipratropium and oxitropium competitively block muscarinic receptors (C). Theophylline inhibits phosphodiesterase (D).

5. D

Chloramphenicol is a broad-spectrum antibiotic used for infections caused by such organisms as *Bacteroides*, *Haemophilus influenzae*, *Neisseria meningitidis*, *Salmonella*, *Rickettsia*, and many vancomycin-resistant enterococci (VREs). The classic complication of chloramphenicol is gray baby syndrome, which occurs in neonates. Neonates are unable to effectively hepatically conjugate chloramphenicol, resulting in toxic serum concentrations of the drug. Abdominal distention, vomiting, cyanosis, and circulatory collapse, collectively termed gray baby syndrome, characterize this toxicity. Sulfonamides can cause fetal kernicterus (A), tetracyclines may cause pigmentation of teeth (B), and mothers taking quinine can develop fetal thrombocytopenia (C).

6. A

Glucose 6-phosphate dehydrogenase (G6PD) deficiency is an X-linked enzymatic disorder of red blood cells that results in a hemolytic syndrome induced by the sudden destruction of older, G6PD-deficient erythrocytes after exposure to drugs with a high redox potential. These drugs include the antimalarial drugs, such as primaquine, and the sulfa drugs, including the sulfonylurea glipizide. Also, fava beans, infections, or metabolic abnormalities may result in hemolytic syndrome. Clinically, symptoms of this disorder result from the development of acute hemolytic anemia and include jaundice, pallor, dark urine, and visceral pain. Indomethacin (B), neomycin (C), and aztreonam (D) do not cause this disorder.

7. A

Aminoglycosides function by inhibiting the 30S ribosomal subunit (A). Tetracyclines inhibit both the 30S and 50S subunit (A and B). Macrolides, clindamycin, chloramphenicol, and the streptogramins all inhibit the 50S ribosomal subunit (B), while the oxazolidinones inhibit the 70S ribosomal subunit (C).

8. B

Methotrexate is a folate antagonist that inhibits dihydrofolate reductase and acts on the S-phase of the cell cycle. The vinca alkaloids, vincristine and vinblastine, act on the M phase (A). The taxols, paclitaxel and docetaxel, act on the G2 and M phase (A and C). The topoisomerase inhibitors, topotecan and etoposide, act on late S and early G2 phase. Remember that all alkylating agents are non-cell cycle specific (D).

9. F

Amitriptyline is a tricyclic antidepressant with serious antimuscarinic side effects including urinary retention, constipation, blurred vision, and dry mouth. Other side effects of this medication include confusion, orthostatic hypotension, and tachycardia. Sertraline (A) is a serotonin-selective reuptake inhibitor (SSRI) with side effects that include serotonin syndrome, decreased libido, and weight change. Thioridazine (B) is a typical antipsychotic that can cause extrapyramidal side effects and potential malignant syndrome. Phenelzine (C) is a monoamine oxidase inhibitor (MAOI) that may be associated with hypertensive crisis and serotonin syndrome. Trazodone (D) is a heterocyclic antidepressant associated with sedation and postural hypotension. Nefazadone (E) is also a heterocyclic antidepressant with side effects that include headache, drowsiness, weakness, and liver toxicity. Erythropoietin (G) induces erythropoiesis and may be associated with headache and an influenza-like syndrome. Metformin (H) is an oral hypoglycemic that may be associated with lactic acidosis. Insulin (I) may produce symptoms similar to those described in the question, but is not taken orally.

10. C

One of the primary complaints of patients taking angiotensin-converting enzyme inhibitors (ACEIs), such as lisinopril, is a chronic, nagging, nonproductive cough that is believed to occur secondary to a drug-induced elevation in circulating bradykinin levels. Generally, these patients can be switched to an angiotensin II receptor blocker (ARB), such as losartan. ARBs have the same clinical efficacy as ACEIs, but with a lower incidence of chronic cough. None of the other answer choices includes chronic cough in their side effect profile.

11. D

Abciximab is an antiplatelet agent used primarily in the setting of cardiac catheterization. This agent acts as a monoclonal antibody directed at the platelet glycoprotein IIb/IIIa receptor, and thereby prevents the binding of fibrinogen and von Willebrand factor. Dipyridamole acts to inhibit platelet adenosine uptake (A) and as a phosphodiesterase inhibitor. Ticlopidine and clopidogrel irreversibly inhibit ADP receptors on platelets (B). Aspirin inhibits prostaglandin production (C).

12. B

Reye's syndrome is an acquired encephalopathy of young children that follows an acute febrile illness, usually influenza or varicella infection, and is characterized by vomiting, agitation, and lethargy, which may progress to coma with intracranial hypertension or death resulting from brain edema and cerebral herniation. This syndrome is strongly associated with aspirin use, and is the reason why aspirin is contraindicated in children. Administration of any of the other drugs listed would not likely result in the described scenario.

13. A

Imipenem is a broad-spectrum carbapenem that acts by inhibiting bacterial transpeptidases and penicillin-binding proteins. This agent is classically associated with CNS toxicity and the development of seizures. Aztreonam is associated with thrombocytopenia (B). Clindamycin is classically associated with pseudomembranous colitis (C) (although a number of antibiotics can cause this). Aminoglycosides are generally associated with ototoxicity (D).

14. C

Patients with the congenital syndrome Wolff-Parkinson-White (WPW) have an additional, or alternative, cardiac pathway, known as an accessory pathway, that directly connects the atria and ventricles, thereby bypassing the AV node. In WPW syndrome, conduction through the bypass tract results in the earlier activation of the ventricles than if the impulse had traveled through the AV node, leading to tachycardia with a short PR interval. Digoxin is not used in these patients because it enhances vagal tone, depressing conduction through the AV node, and it increases the risk of conduction via the accessory pathway. The other drugs mentioned do not influence cardiac conduction.

15. B

Omeprazol binds irreversibly to the H^+/K^+-ATPase pump in parietal cells. In order for parietal cells to overcome this inhibition, they must synthesize entirely new H^+/K^+-ATPase proteins, which typically takes about 24 hours.

16. B

SVT is an arrhythmia that originates in myocardial tissue above the ventricles, either in atrial and/or atrioventricular (AV) junctional tissue. SVT is commonly described as a narrow QRS complex tachycardia, because conduction remains normal through the ventricles (by way of the Purkinje fibers). The agents of choice to treat this arrhythmia, propranolol or verapamil, act by slowing conduction velocity through the AV node, resulting in a decreased ventricular rate.

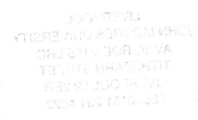

17. C

Loperamide is an antidiarrheal agent that acts by activating presynaptic opioid receptors in the enteric nervous system, inhibiting peristalsis and prolonging fecal transit time. Kaolin, pectin, and methylcellulose are all antimotility agents that act by adsorbing intestinal toxins and micro-organisms (A), thereby protecting the intestinal mucosa and increasing stool viscosity. Misoprostol is a prostaglandin E_1 analog (B) used in patients with peptic ulcer disease and has no use for reducing diarrhea.

18. D

Any patient taking metronidazole should be warned against the concurrent ingestion of alcohol because of a subsequent disulfiram-like reaction that presents clinically as flushing, nausea, chest palpitations and pain, vertigo, and hypotension. Cheese (A) is contraindicated while taking MAOIs (phenelzine and tranylcypromine). Milk (B) is not an absolute contraindication for most medications. Aspirin (C) is contraindicated in children because of Reye's syndrome.

19. C

During pregnancy, heparin can be safely used in pregnant mothers. Urokinase (A) is an acute thrombolytic that would not be used as a chronic anticoagulant. Warfarin (B) is a teratogen associated with nasal hypoplasia, optic atrophy, microcephaly, and mental retardation and is con-traindicated in pregnancy.

20. A

Warfarin is an anticoagulant that inhibits vitamin K epoxide reductase, thereby preventing the formation of clotting factors II, VII, IX, and X. Warfarin is cleared hepatically by the cytochrome P-450 system and is subject to alterations in its rate of clearance by other medications that induce or inhibit on the P-450 system. Amiodarone (A), quinidine, chloramphenicol, ketoconazole, ranitidine, verapamil, isoniazid, ciprofloxacin, cimetidine, and erythromycin all inhibit P-450 and may result in elevated plasma levels of hepatically cleared medications. Inducers of P-450, which would decrease plasma levels of hepatically cleared agents, include griseofulvin (B), phenobarbital (C), carbamazepine (D), alcohol, rifampin, and phenytoin.

21. H

1% to 2% of patients taking statins, such as simvastatin, experience an elevation in liver enzymes. None of the other answers listed significantly elevates liver enzymes.

22. D

Ciprofloxacin is contraindicated in pregnant women, infants, and children because of potential problems with connective tissue development. The other medications listed are not contraindi-cated in children.

23. D

Recognize that this molecule contains a β-lactam ring. The possibility exists that β-lactamase-producing bacterium capable of hydrolyzing site D would be resistant to the new drug's effects.

24. C

Recall that the half-life ($T_{1/2}$) is the time required for the concentration of the drug to drop by 50% in a reference body fluid, in this case the blood. The question states that the initial concen-tration of the drug in the blood is 1 mg/L. Following one $T_{1/2}$, the concentration of the drug in the blood will be 0.5 mg/L. In order for the concentration of the drug to drop to 0.25 mg/L ($^1/_4$ of it original concentration), it will require two half-lives ($^1/_2 \times {}^1/_2 = {}^1/_4$). The $T_{1/2}$ of the drug can be calculated using the formula: $T_{1/2} = 0.69 \times$ volume of distribution (mL) / clearance (mL/hour). The clearance of the drug is given as 100 mL/hour. The volume of distribution of the drug can be calculated using the following formula: volume of distribution = dose (mg)/initial plasma concentration (mg/mL). The calculated VD is 5000 mL. Plugging these values into the formula for $T_{1/2}$ results in a value of 34.5 hours. Thus, the concentration of the drug in the plasma will drop by 50% in 34.5 hours. The concentration of the drug will drop to 25% of its original level in 69 hours (C).

25. A

Recall that a physiologic antagonist is one that produces antagonism stimulating a receptor and producing an effect that is opposite to the effect of another agonist acting at a separate receptor. The only choice that fits this definition is answer A. Stimulation of α-adrenergic receptors results in contraction of radial muscles of the iris and dilation of the pupil. This effect would antagonize the contraction of the pupils induced by carbachol. Answer B describes a pharmacologic, or recep-tor, antagonist. Answer C describes a chemical antagonist. Answer D describes a dispositional, or pharmacokinetic, antagonist.

Index

Index note: page references with a *b*, *f*, or *t* indicate a box, figure, or table on the designated page; page references in **bold** indicate discussion of the subject in the Hardcore Figures and Graphs or Practice Questions and Answers section.